HEALTH OR HELL

…Choice is yours

Dr. Rajasekhar Ramakrishna Mysore

STARDOM BOOKS

STARDOM BOOKS

WORLDWIDE

www.StardomBooks.com

STARDOM BOOKS

A Division of Stardom Publishing

and infoYOGIS Technologies.

105-501 Silverside Road

Wilmington, DE 19809

FIRST EDITION OCTOBER 2020

Stardom Books

HEALTH OR HELL

…Choice is yours

Dr. Rajasekhar Ramakrishna Mysore

p. 186
cm. 13.5 X 21.5

Category: HEALTH & FITNESS / SELF-HELP / Holism

ISBN-13: 978-1-7332116-7-3

The book just happened.

But the choice of the right person to write the foreword was daunting.

Who's the best person to judge the book on its merit, and how is he qualified?

Again it happened.

Who can be a better judge than the **honorable former Chief Justice of The Supreme Court of India**?

What better way to qualify than being a living legend in his 10th decade of perfect health? A learned person who headed the National Human Rights Commission, National Commission to review the working of the Constitution of India, Chairman of Ethical guidelines for Biogenetic research of Indian Council of Medical Research, etc. to name a few?

He is none other than **Sri M.N.VENKATACHALIAH**. A great human being who is difficult to emulate.

Thanking him is too small an effort. This great personality blesses me and the book. I am overwhelmed.

Also, I owe it to Sri P.V. Ravishanker, who took a lot of pains in this regard. I am obliged to him.

FOREWORD

The only justification for this invitation for an extraneous 'Foreword' to an excellent medical treatise is not to seek. I was a friend of the author's father, Sri Ramakrishna, a leading and successful lawyer who studied law under my father.

Though subtle humour permeates the text and the narrative, Dr. Rajasekhar deals with some serious health and disease aspects. Good health is not the mere absence of illness and disease. It is much more. It is the expression of the neuro-humoral, neuro-endocrinal, neuro-hormonal homeostasis. The mind has much to do with this.

In an interesting study on life expectancy and aging, Ray Kurzweil and Dr. Terry Grossman examine and dispel some popular assumptions of limits of human life-span, aging, and deaths. They say:

"Most of our conceptions of human-life in
the 21st Century will be turned on their head.
Not the least of these is the expectation
expressed in the adage about the inevitability
of death and taxes. We will leave the issue of
the future of taxes to another book. But
belief in the inevitability of death and how this
perspective will soon change is very much the
primary theme of this Book".

"Fantastic Voyage" P.4

Human life-span extension scientist Aubrey De Grey in his "Engineered Negligible Senescence: Rational Design of feasible, Comprehensive Rejuvenation Bio-Technology," speaks of the potential for infinite expansion of human life-span. But how does man manage the vast expansion of his life-span when he does not even know how to spend a rainy Sunday afternoon usefully! Noble purpose in life alone justifies longevity.

Dr. Rajasekhar's "Health or Hell" gives some good-news and useful tips for great health and happiness. Doctors like him are assets of the society we live in. They are gifts from God. May God bless him with long life and great health.

M.N. Venkatachaliah
Bangalore
November 1, 2020

PRAISE FOR THE BOOK

Happy to know my good friend – Dr. Rajasekhar Mysore, has authored his first book on Health for lay man and professional colleagues.

He is the first writer who called the readers of the book as "authors". I am amazed to note the flow of thoughts, the format of writing, particularly nectar and beacons. This is definitely "Do it yourself" and "see it yourself" kind of book.

The author's way of breaking myths on health is the need of the hour. The examples quoted in the book are from the author's vast medical experience, wide travelling and meditation is appreciable.

Overall it is a very good venture. I am sure this is the beginning of much more to come from him. Wish you all the best.

Dr. Anjanappa T M
Medical director, Mamatha nursing home
& Former Medical Superintendent at KIMS, Bengaluru

DEDICATION

I want to dedicate this book to all the great souls I have come across in my personal and professional life, the ilks of Chandrika, Shruthi, Parimala, Geeta, and Sonal. These women succeeded in overcoming their rare, devastating, life-threatening diseases at the beginning and peak of their careers with sheer indomitable spirit and grit.

Also,

- To the medical fraternity, who knows everything about disease and treatment, but little about health.
- To those individuals who work for others' health, neglecting their own.
- To those who advise people with good intentions, without practicing them.
- To those innocent intellectuals, who believe that medical science is pure science and follow it religiously.
- To those paramedical and pseudo-medical professionals who believe and make others think that they know all about health.

.

ACKNOWLEDGEMENTS

I thank all those who knowingly or unknowingly, with good or bad intentions, wholeheartedly, or half-heartedly supported me in this endeavor.
I acknowledge the troubles caused by me while writing this book to my patients, my staff, my colleagues, and my family members - who have not expressed their displeasure or resentment and were extremely patient with me.
Special thanks to
Malathi Venugopal for designing the cover page and other artwork in the book. Many thanks to Manaswini, Prithvija, for helping me compile all the material. Thank you, Raam Anand and team for making the process of writing the book enjoyable.
Many thanks to the unknown and the unknowable, for making this happen.

CHARITI

"Diseases do not discriminate between rich and poor! So should the treatment."

With this goal in mind, 'CHARITI,' the charitable wing of Chirag Hospital, has charted out the following.

1. To reduce the burden of diseases, Health should be promoted by educating people about prioritizing health and how to go about it.
2. Innovative technologies in medical diagnosis and treatment are accessible to all.
3. Financial help for treatment.

This book is part of the first goal, and the financial returns will go to CHARITI for furthering this noble cause. By reading this book, you are not only getting health benefits, but you also get to be a partner of CHARITI.

CONTENTS

PART A

PART B

PART C

PREFACE

"Corona Virus and coronary disease, what the hell???"
What is hell?
My grandmother used to tell that when one dies, if they go
to hell, that person will be subjected to torture like poking,
cutting, burning, etc. But, I always used to think, when a body
is buried or burnt, how can they do that? But, now I
understand those things are possible in this world only...in the
form of diseases and their management. "So, Hell is here!"
"CHOICE IS YOURS!"

There are:

- N number of diseases (N is in thousands) – named and
unnamed.
- N^2 solutions – magical, religious, home remedies, traditional,
alternative, natural, modern, scientific, etc.
- N^3 experts – hardly anybody who will not advise on the
treatment of any disease.
- N^4 dilemmas – which one to choose, when, where, what,
how, side effects, after effects, expenses, opinions – 2nd, 3rd...
advertisements, unsolicited advice.
YOU, the intelligent, hardworking, ambitious, and time-
poor individual, has to deal with all these before embarking on
any treatment, none of which are fail-proof. So, there is a need
to get clarity and make the right decisions at the right time and
at the right place, all of which have to be decided by YOU.
This is not another book on health tips, like, - what to eat

1

and when, what sort of exercises, how much to sleep, etc. There are many such books out there. You can use them with a purpose, once you have clarity.

This book is neither for those who outsource their health to god or fate nor for those who offer themselves to an AMC (Annual Maintenance Contract) at hospitals and diagnostic centers.

This book is for YOU, who believes that health is not just wealth, but Everything. And, for those who want to remain healthy without wasting money, time, or effort, on their own.

It is a self-assessment type of book, where you will answer FAQs asked by most of you to a doctor. Go through the chapters and at the end of the book, answer those questions, and evaluate yourself.

The examples quoted are real-life stories from my practice and suggestions given from my own true-life experiences. After experiencing this book, you will become happy, healthy, and whole

MEET THE WRITER

Hello! Dear Reader, I am so happy that you've chosen this book. Before we go on this ruminating journey, let me tell you a little about myself, Mysore Ramakrishna Rajasekhar, a practicing surgeon and proctologist.

My professional identity as a Doctor, in my personal opinion, is as follows:

It's my destiny to become a Doctor, to tinker with the human bodies and emotions. With more ignorance than knowledge at hand, I am expected to give the hapless fellow human beings relief from their sufferings. My patients trust me so much by offering their most complex and precious gadget, the body, which is restituted by chemicals, cutting, stitching, welding, and even removing parts. They put me on a divine high pedestal delicately supported by my wobbling expertise but somehow held together by 'His' gracious support. With the patient's trust, affection, and overbearing expectations — probably in no other profession can one enjoy the fascination of ignorance, the bliss.

Now let's get to 'why we need this book on health?'

In the 46 years that I have spent in the medical field, I have witnessed the paradigm shift that has taken place in the diagnosis and treatment of diseases. The sophistication, accuracy, safety in the practice of modern medicine today is phenomenal.

However, with the foray of all branches of sciences, media, legalities, and commerce into the medical practice, we lost the plot. We were led to believe that technology is the only solution and suffice to be legally correct.

Our end goal was to banish diseases while our means were science and numbers. We forgot that the pivotal point of all our efforts was to maintain the health of fellow human beings. We became focused on statistics and publications. This became the evidence that we held on to, as gospel truth, without giving much thought to its insufficiency or negative effect.

Likewise, the elements of common sense and trust began to erode, and the process of treating patients became more technical than pragmatic and compassionate.

Furthermore, treatment became convoluted because we relied on elaborate scientific means and protocols as opposed to using simple, practical methods.

What's worse is that these methods have been counterproductive in the long run because our approach was disease-centric, technology-oriented, and market-driven, and not so much about wellness and people's health.

With this framework in place, the gap between rich and poor in regards to healthcare facilities further widened. The focus shifted to the commercialization of medical facilities.

On one hand, we've eradicated smallpox and a host of other diseases. Still, on the other, we have found ourselves devastated by lifestyle-related diseases like diabetes, cardiac diseases, and obesity. These lifestyle-diseases are essentially a product of the mindset of indulgence, consumerism, and false notions.

No section of the population was spared — the rich acquired indulgence and arrogance, like obesity, addictions, and mental disorders. The middle class tried to ape the rich. Then these diseases trickled down to the middle-class and the poor. While the rich have various avenues and treatment options, the middle class and the poor have to run from pillar to post to make ends meet. The poor became more impoverished due to illness.

Furthermore, the way doctors approach health today needs to change. The focus must be on wellness, preventing, and reversing disorders. Sure, science is the solution, but it is not the final and the only answer.

Why can't we approach other methods? Why can't it be individualistic? Health is not the responsibility of doctors. It is the responsibility of us individuals. Health can't be outsourced to the medical profession.

These were the questions disturbing me. Then I realized why not talk to my patients directly as a friend and explain to them. I am particularly troubled by the way patients look at doctors as a last resort, a necessary evil!

Individuals must be empowered to take care of their health. My main goal here is to promote individual health consciousness so that they are able to prevent lifestyle diseases.

This is a 'Do It Yourself' and a 'See It Yourself' book, which will help you get your health back. In all the chaos, you're hard-pressed for time and confused in regards to making a decision. You need clarity.

If your next question is, what will this book do for me? Here are the answers.

- This book is like a little workbook for introspection. You can even call it a passbook for serial entries on your well-being.
- It could be a cookbook to help you prepare delicacies of peace and happiness.
- It could be a logbook where you can learn from your mistakes.
- It might as well be a cheque book for you to encash the benefits of realization.

Here's How You Can Read This Book:

Those of you who want to read leisurely, understand the whole process of health, and get full benefits, start from front cover to the end and enjoy every bit of it.

Don't rush through the book. Read one chapter at a time, understand, contemplate, and write down any doubts and answer the questions at the end of chapters.

Please go through the 'Nectar' and 'Beacons' towards the end of the book and try to familiarize yourself with the concept. Try to practice the tips and tricks so that you can get the most out of this book and make a lasting change.

Those of you who are hard-pressed for time can start from the back cover. Go through the 'Beacons' and the diagrams for a quick procurement of knowledge.

Those who have 'no time' can open the page no 143, recite and repeat the 'mantra' mentioned, with full concentration and feeling, to get some benefits.

The primary purpose of this book is to transform the way we look at health.

PART A

PROLOGUE

MY STORY – MYSTERY TO MASTERY

I

Long long ago, more than 5000 days back, on an unusually dull day, there was a phone call that changed the course of my life and shifted my focus. Seated on a comfortable chair behind my desk, after a heavy breakfast, I struggled to keep awake as I waited for patients in the OPD of our new nursing home. I was listening to a pleasantly divine composition. I'm guessing by A. R. Rahman. That's when I heard a voice in my head. It was a sentence, I think, from God himself.

"The whole world is healthy, so you relax. Enjoy the music."

"What?" I replied. "I have to face the music if there are no patients."

My reverie was interrupted by a voice from reality. "Saar, your phone has been ringing for a long time now," said the Ayah. "I know," I replied, feigning awareness. "I was meditating, and as always, you've disturbed me."

I looked at my phone and saw three missed calls. Those were the days when missed calls were used as a mode of communication, as the call charges were exorbitant. I avoided calls from unknown numbers unless they were too many within a short time interval, indicating some emergency. Anyhow, I decided to ring back, expecting to hear from a patient complaining of postoperative pain. A few rings later, I heard a vaguely familiar voice.

9

It was not of a patient. It was a remotely familiar voice generating a feeling of pleasantness inside me. "Sekhar, can you hear me? It's me, Raja. Your classmate from the 7th class at Penukonda. I hope you remember me. You're a big man now. Busy? I hope I am not disturbing you." There was some disturbance, and all I did was mutter a hello and tried to recognize the voice.

When I finally heard, "Hey, Source... It's me, Resource..." The phone went dead. The Ayah, with her characteristic smile, brought the charger and asked me to connect it to the nearest plug point. A face flashed before my eyes, and I went back in time.

I was in Class 7. It was Independence Day, 1968, and I was in the field watching the headmaster as he stood before a giant pole on top of which the National flag was tied. He was ready to unfurl the flag when suddenly there was a commotion; a giant monkey was spotted at the scene. He seemed to have a shoe in his hand, which belonged to the headmaster. The monkey was quickly climbing up the pole, while the PT teacher tried to scare him and get him to drop the shoe but to no avail.

Amid the chaos, a puny little boy started climbing the pole behind the monkey. Teachers were stunned, and children were watching eagerly with gaping mouths, fearing that the monkey would attack him. He slowly took out a handful of peanuts from his pocket and gave it to the monkey in exchange for the shoe! Nobody knew who he was, as he had just joined the school after his father got transferred to our town. There was jubilation all around.

Raja! I could feel myself smiling. Just then, I received a call from him again, and we chatted a bit about our little adventures. He told me he had found a new job in the city and wanted to meet me. We agreed to meet soon for our usual *Resource Vs. Source* session.

RESOURCE VS SOURCE?

On the night of the Independence Day celebration, Raja

came to my house with his father to borrow some notes that the teacher had given in the previous months. Raja was joining the school in the middle of the term. I was famous as the student who came first in class. So, it was not unusual for his father to ask for my notes. I gave Raja the notes. Albeit not all because I loved my first rank too much to share it with anyone else. Anyway, my fears were unwarranted because he didn't want my notes at all. He was only there because his father had asked him to do so.

All Raja cared about was studying from guides and passing exams, while for me, even a second rank in a single subject was unacceptable. We became good friends quickly, as we were poles apart. We would often go on long walks and talk about things. That's when I learned that Raja was a street-smart kid with quick-fix solutions to all situations in life. He was resourceful, and the teachers loved him for that, but his father thought he was good for nothing. This upset Raja, even if it wasn't true. He was good at solving problems, and what he couldn't do, he would delegate. He would outsource solving analytical problems and passing exams to me. Because he was resourceful and I was the source of answers, I called him Resource, and he called me Source. These were our nicknames for each other.

One day, I was explaining Newton's Laws of Motion to him, he exclaimed, "What? Laws of motion? I know them. Daily morning, I use them in the loo, the more pressure you apply…" "Shut up!" I yelled. "Regular versus loose motions," he shouted and ran away.

The next day, after the phone call, Raja and I met at a restaurant that sold what was known as "Single Idly and by-two coffee" and nicknamed, "SIDBYTCO!"

Resource arrived and quickly recognized me. I, on the other hand, took my time because he had replaced his lean body and curly hair with a cushion of fat and a receding hairline. He had begun talking about himself and filling me up on what happened in his life.

He told me that he joined a multinational company as an IT Professional once he finished his graduation in Commerce. He said he was getting paid more than what he was worth. All he had to do was work a little longer and consider sleep a waste of time. He told me that his motto was work is worship, and he kept going up the corporate ladder with fancy titles like team leader and regional manager. Not just that, he had complementary titles to those that he had achieved. They were diabetic, hypertensive, sleep-disordered, and whatnot.

The newest title was coronary artery disease with angioplasty as the treatment option and working from home. This bewildered him, and he decided to visit me. He was now a part of the group of corporate administrators who coined humane phrases like 'waiting on the bench,' 'work from home,' 'golden shake hand,' VRS, Pink slips, etc., to announce impending disasters for their employees!

Needless to say, he was stressed and had loans to repay. So quitting wasn't an option. He added that he didn't have the time to smoke, drink, and wasn't even a fan of eating out. He joined the gym and did a bit of yoga. He read health books and magazines cover to cover, and got himself regular health check-ups. He had an impressive insurance package paid for by the company.

Occasionally, he visited a resort or joined a laughter club to relax. He did everything he could do to stay healthy and yet ended up with a list of illnesses. "Why are these diseases so fond of me?" He asked me with fear in his eyes even as he tried to make light of the situation. Then, as if trying to console me, he told me he had a two-million-rupees-insurance.

"Tell me what should I do?" He asked. "Also, take 'your week' to answer," he ludicrously reminded me of our time in the past where he would come up to me with deep questions, and I'd take a week to respond to them.

"I won't waste time," I said. "You and I will sit together, and you'll listen to me. You'll follow what I tell you. I can't lose any more wickets!" I almost yelled. After losing two classmates in three months to cardiac arrest, I had become over-sensitive to humor on health. To my surprise, Resource agreed to the plan with a smile.

"Alright," he said. "For the next seven weeks, I will bring a question every week, and you work on it. At the end of the sessions, there should be a solution to all my health problems."

"This whole thing will be a discussion," I replied. "Even though I can treat illness, I want to empower you to know about your health and reverse lifestyle diseases." I insisted that he ask questions and not just nod to my methods.

At first, I meticulously took down his medical history. Everything seemed okay. He initially took one tablet for diabetes and then moved up to two, three, and so on; now, he needs insulin.

I found that all his diseases had aggravated with time. I got him to talk about his lifestyle to get a peek into his routine and philosophy. I was getting somewhere with all this information.

That is when he blurted out as a matter of factly, "You doctors don't know how to stop a disease or reverse it. It keeps progressing, and all you do is add newer treatments." I was quiet. I didn't have an answer to that.

II

Before my next meeting with Resource, I did my homework and thought about what I would tell him. I dissected out his whole story. What is the conclusion?

I started by saying we all must know answers for two basic questions.

1. Who am I?
2. What is life?

He was perplexed. So, I started explaining why these questions are important for health, "Picture this out. You have joined a new company for your job. The very first day, you noticed some commotion at the entrance; some employees are shouting at one another. You pacified them and settled the issue. The next day, there was a problem with the computer in the front office. You tried your hand at it. It worked. The next day, an electric problem, you solved that as well.

When, in fact, you are a Commerce graduate and have nothing to do with those things. The following day, you tried to interfere in a fight. It escalated, and this annoyed the boss. When you tried to fix a problem on the computer, it crashed. The boss was furious. Your attempt to correct an electrical issue resulted in a small blast. Your boss summoned you."

"Who are you? Why are you meddling with everything?"

"Sir, please tell me, WHO AM I in this organization? I will take up my responsibilities accordingly. You were then sent to the accounts department, asked to sort out files, and forward them to different departments.

You started your work earnestly, and a copy of all the documents was forwarded by you to IT, thinking that it is the Information & Technology department. Alas, the Income Tax department came for an inspection!"

You must know what an organization is about when you become a part of it. Similarly, in the organization of life, you must know 'Who you are?' and 'What is life?'

"What's my fault in this?" Resource asked me. "I followed all the advice given to me by the doctor at the company. I followed all the preventive measures and got regular health checkups."

He then went on to tell me about his company doctor. "He's a nice guy, but I often find him in the smoking zones. I know it's a personal matter, but I asked him anyway If he was stressed or something. After all, why would he smoke despite the

14

warnings."

I remember him chuckling and asking me, "Do I look perturbed?" The doctor then continued, "I was in the army and had a great job. There was respect and regard. I was the boss. Post-retirement, I couldn't adjust to private practice.

I was seen as strict and vain by my colleagues and patients. So, I joined here for the package and perks. I mean, the work is easy, and all I have to do is deal with IDIOT patients. Sure, professional satisfaction is low, but I'm making do."

Looking at my dismayed expression, the doctor clarified, "IDIOT is an acronym for 'Internet Derived Information Obstructing Treatment.'

I thought you're familiar with this acronym." In response to my smile, the doctor continued narrating his predicament. "You see, I get bored a lot, and whenever that happens, I step out for six or seven cigarettes." "Much more," I corrected. "My wife is annoyed at my new habit, so I finish my weekly quota at work. Weekends are hard. I have become a cigarette connoisseur," the doctor laughed. "I refrained from saying anything to the doctor because it was his personal matter." Concluded Resource.

"But can a doctor who smokes convince his patients about the ill effects of smoking?" I wondered.

Resource nodded and summarized, "As I understand, I followed all the so-called precautions advised by my doctor without understanding how life works.

I went on accumulating disease after disease, thinking that I had no choice and accepting it as a part of my corporate gift."

Resource's medicines were medically correct, and we talked about his habits and life-philosophy.

Armed with this knowledge, I began meditating on health. I define meditation as giving serious and careful thought to a topic without the self at the centre. My little method has seven sages. They comprise the crux of this book. They are as follows:

1. What?

2. Why?
3. How?
4. When?
5. Who?
6. Where?
7. Which?

SAGE 1
WHAT IS HEALTH?

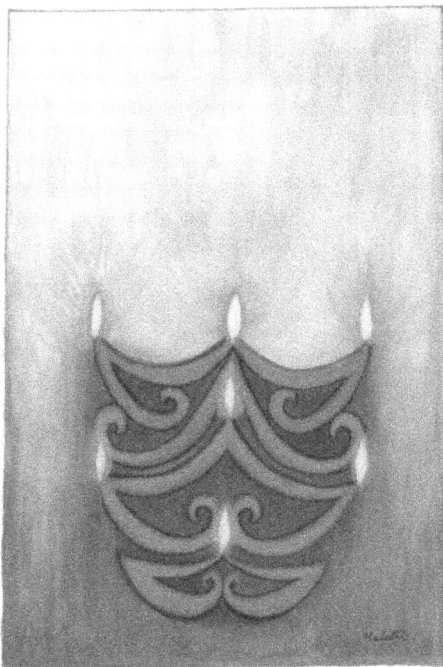

Intending to solve Resource's problem, the two of us sat down like we used to, back in the day, where he would come up to me with a question, and I would take a week to get back to him.

The first question was, what is health. But here's how

Resource put it out for me. "Why did I get all these diseases?"

This is perhaps the most common question a doctor encounters if the patients are allowed to ask questions. The second I heard the question, my brain had begun comprehending it and breaking it down.

I divided my friend's question into three parts. What is disease? Why did he get it? Why does anyone get it?

If I have to rely on my conventional medical wisdom, then I would pin it down to the etiological or the idiopathic factors that lead to a person developing a disease. It would be easy for me to use my professional jargon to help him understand. But, I think that approach doesn't help. I am aware that my knowledge is by no means unlimited.

All professionals use jargon to confuse the listener and to appear intellectual. For instance, a doctor prefers to say hemorrhoids instead of piles, and legal luminaries say '*res ipsa loquitur*' instead of, the thing speaks for itself. The priests have the advantage of Sanskrit, Arabic, Biblical English, or Hebrew when cornered. The use of Greek and Latin merely masks our ignorance and limited knowledge of the subject. Of course, it adds glamour to our intellectual aura!

With this presupposition, let me now explain to you what a disease is.

DISEASE

A disease is an impairment in the parameters of the physical and chemical processes of the body. It manifests as an illness by feelings in our minds. When the parameters change, and there is decreased physical and mental energy, it is termed as sickness.

HEALTH

Now, the dictionary definition of health is the condition of being sound in body, mind, or spirit. Oftentimes, it is seen as a goal as opposed to a lifestyle. Health is an expression of life.

Life comprises four components that work in conjunction with each other. The processes are physical processes, chemical reactions, energy generation and distribution, and intelligence.

PHYSICAL PROCESS

The hardware part of life structure is the body, consisting of organs, tissues, cells, enwrapped by skin, including the skin.

The disturbances in this hardware can be from injury, deformity, lump/swelling, discoloration, variations in quantity like size, weight, etc. The body is the most easily identifiable part of the human structure. So, we easily identify with that as 'me.' Though it is only a hardware part, we give more importance to it. The attachment to it causes emotional perversions like pride, discrimination, possessiveness, anger, frustration, etc.

A computer is identified with its operating system rather than with hardware Windows 2000 /XP, DOS, LINUX, etc. not with the screen, monitor, keyboard, mouse et al. So should our identity be expressed with our operating system -- the inner energy. I still remember Akash, that fitness freak with a 6-pack-abdomen, got admitted to a major corporate hospital for Gastroenteritis, which causes loose stools, vomiting, and dehydration. He was shaking.

He feared that he'd die, so he called and texted everyone he knew and requested them to pray for him. He apologized to the folks he had bullied. Eventually, he got better and learned that physical strength is not everything. My point here is that focusing on brawn alone will not help you. By all means, make sure you exercise and stay healthy but don't think that it's all you have to do. Physical fitness is only a part of overall good health.

CHEMICAL PROCESS

You are hungry, and you see your favorite food in front of you. You get the nice smell of it, a chemical process. You start eating it, saliva is dripping, a chemical process. Food reaches the stomach, digestive juices are secreted, a chemical process. It goes on...that way. All activities in, through, and by the body are chemically mediated, including the process of digestion, metabolism, excretion, neurological signal transmission, including thinking processes, emotions, etc. Every single cell is a chemical factory.

The nucleus inside the cell is its head office consisting of chromosomes, genes, DNA, etc. It interacts with the outer components inside the cell through chemical mediators. The cell wall is made of hundreds of gates called receptors, which allow only specific chemicals in and out through them. Many require gate passes, which are also chemicals. For example, if glucose, which is the essential source of energy, has to enter the cell, it requires a chemical called insulin to open the gate called insulin receptor present on every cell.

Each living cell is not only a factory but a world by itself. The activities, intentions, emotions are no less than those of the whole universe, though on a miniature scale. The body has the innate capacity to manufacture all the required chemicals, and the ingredients come from outside through oral, nasal, or dermal routes or artificially through injections. The waste products are excreted to keep the chemicals balanced, through urine, motions, sweat, or vomitus, etc. Signals like hunger/satiety regulate the need for required ingredients; appetite/aversion; taste, smell, flavors through sensors in the mouth, tongue, nose, stomach, etc., contribute to the same. It is not uncommon to see people after overeating asking for digestive enzymes so that they will be ready for the next meal on time! The chemicals introduced into the body as medicines, stimulants like alcohol, nicotine, drugs, etc. have repercussions on the whole system.

ENERGY GENERATION & DISTRIBUTION

Our internal energy, which provides us with enthusiasm, creativity, confidence, etc., is part of the cosmic energy. It gets recharged during rest, sleep, and meditation. This energy also has to be conserved by avoiding uncalled for, unnecessary, unproductive, and purposeless actions, which will dissipate all the energies.

Gurunath, an upcoming young musician, very active and energetic, came to my clinic with complaints of losing weight for the past six months, feeling exhausted in spite of nutrient supplements. A battery of tests was ordered. All the tests were within normal limits. It was the season for music nights and fests. He was worried that his budding career may be ruined. Many specialists were consulted. At last, the full-body CT scan revealed a cyst in the brain. The culprit was caught. All arrangements were readied for the neurosurgery. At the time of giving consent, he noticed a term that there is a possibility of damage to the speech area during the procedure. He refused surgery and came to me for opinion, as his father was my friend. My initial suspicion was some hidden cancer somewhere. I went through all his records carefully—nothing to suggest anything amiss. Before raising my hands up in despair, I just started inquiring about his routine, just to buy time to get some more ideas.

He told me he wakes up around 9 am, takes a cup of coffee, gets ready, and goes to work by 10 am. Students will be ready for training. Finishes the first session by 1 pm. He then has his brunch. The second session is between 2 pm to 5 pm, followed by coffee. The third session is between 5 pm to 9 pm. Post that dinner and tea. Between 10 pm to 4 am, he composes music, as it is quiet then, and he gets many ideas. He also smokes a few cigarettes at that time to get his brain working. He did not remember when he went to bed because most of the time, he would have fallen asleep in his seat. I had an intuition that this has something to do with his weight loss. I suggested that he come for yoga therapy at my center for 3 hours a day. It was divided into 1 hour of exercise, 1-hour meditation, and 1-hour sleep. For 3 weeks, he attended and felt much better.

I asked him to gradually reduce yoga and meditation from his schedule and continue to sleep for an hour or so in the afternoon. I told him sleep is not falling dead by exhaustion. It is a process for recharging your energies. Sleep is not a waste of time. I used yoga and meditation just to attract him to sleep as a therapy. He regained his appetite and weight and improved his efficiency.

"So, sleep is not a passive phase but an essential one;

definitely not a waste of time. The cyst in his brain was only an incidental finding. It had nothing to do with his symptoms!" Resource remarked. "Exactly, in fact, sleep has more benefits besides recharging," I added.

Why do you think some people are energetic, and some are a little low? Let me explain, energy gets utilized in the physical and chemical processes. Imagine a smartphone with too many background apps open throughout the day. Its battery runs out fast, and you have to recharge it again to make it work. Likewise, if you're someone who thinks a lot and worries about everything, you will be fatigued throughout the day, and you need to rest to recharge.

Without breaks and enough sleep, your mind will function slowly and erratically. Furthermore, with unregulated thoughts, your brain is working twice as hard to focus and complete the task at hand. Think of these thoughts as apps open in the background in a phone. They use up all the power quickly, and you're left with a low charge when you have to make that important call. The inner energy that we explored earlier is mental energy. When it begins to deplete, you experience fatigue, frustration, anger, depression, etc. If we understand this concept properly and implement it, then we can prevent emotional outbursts and have better mental health.

INTELLIGENCE

This is our fourth and crucial component of health. It is a guiding principle for us humans. It is composed of four factors. They are innate intelligence, intellect, mind, and memories.

1. Innate intelligence:

It is pervading through all cells, tissues, and organs; and runs that machinery in subconscious mode. This is the original software downloaded as an operating system. This one is essential for all our biological living. This innate intelligence guides all the regular clockwork-like, minute-to-minute activities occurring inside the body. We are not even aware of this, and so we take it for granted. The other high-profile components of intelligence, like intellect and memory, are more appreciated. As innate intelligence is all-pervasive in each cell and organ, the disturbance in this component affects the whole system and results in the so-called lifestyle diseases. This being ubiquitous and very subtle, is beyond the reach of even intellect. So, manipulating this by medical or surgical means yields very erratic and at the most temporary results.

'Placebo effect,' 'faith-healing,' 'good healing hand' are some of the effects that occur through this energy. Black magic, curse, grace, astrological solutions, etc. probably act through this energy. It is in constant communication with all-pervasive, universal cosmic energy.

This being the equivalent of the original OS, it should be kept away from malware, viruses, worms, etc., and constantly renewed and upgraded. This part of intelligence does not identify with the body and has no attachment to the concept of me, mine, my, etc.

2. Intellect:

It is the analyzing and filtering tool of intelligence, to categorize thoughts into useful or useless, important or not, productive or unproductive. It is judgemental and helps in taking decisions or directions in day to day life. This is the most celebrated part of intelligence—people who are respected as highly intellectual use its analytical power and speed well.

Intellect has its own limitations. It can only compute and analyze and conclude only from the available information in mind, that too, when it is not disturbed by emotions. We believe that two heads are better than one. Many times, it is not so. Now with more and more information at our fingertips, thanks to the internet and mobile phone, making decisions for intellect has become an arduous task. It leaves us more confused with multiple options, even for a simple problem. Intellect also has the limitation of the logic it has learned, for it can act only through it. *Let me tell you a story of Kamala, 87, who was bed-ridden due to paralysis for three months. Her two sons were doctors, and one of them retired early to care for her. She had developed a fever and was losing weight quickly, so she was being treated in the ICU for about two months, but the improvement was little. She had to be taken home and required round-the-clock care. Now, my opinion as a human was to keep her at home and take care of her necessities, rather than repeated interventions, which was unpalatable to the son. To my mind, just because we had so many options available did not mean we had to use them on her. Her sons, who were doctors, had to play the role of attendants, and this was hard on them. We ought to use medical knowledge judiciously while also considering the dignity of the patient.*

Also, our emotions affect our intellect, especially in the cases where our loved ones are in pain. However, that can do more damage than good. It's crucial that we operate from a calm and detached mind.

"The intellect is overwhelmed by too much knowledge and stifled with emotions. It should be independent and free of emotions, like the judiciary," Resource added.

The main purpose of INTELLECT is to search and download the appropriate knowledge sites from the universally spread intelligence by contemplation or meditation.

3. Mind:

Receives information through different senses, accumulates, organizes them, interacts with intellect, identifies and discriminates as mine and others, it releases this data as thoughts or commands for action. These thoughts tagged to the identity of 'ME, MINE, MY,' become emotional thoughts and can result in likes/dislikes, love/hatred, enjoy / suffering, success/failure, gain/loss, appreciation/jealousy, etc. The negative ones are the cause of distress to us and those around us.

Generally, emotions are categorized into 6 basic groups and given below are each emotion with the ascending order of their intensity:

1. Wishes, Desires, Wants, Passions, Ambitions, avarice….
2. Disagreement, Frustrations, Anger, Fury, destructive...
3. Saving, not sharing, not using(miserly), hoarding…
4. Likes, love, Attachment, Possessiveness, Lust
5. Pride, discrimination, Arrogance…
6. Inadequacy, jealousy, intolerance...

To make it simple, the emotion of 'wishes' becomes 'desires' and progresses to 'wants' and then to 'passions,' 'ambitions', and finally to 'avarice,' which can result in disasters.

Basic emotions are a part of the formation and sustenance of groups like family, friends, societies, communities, nationalities. These groups are formed by identifying commonalities.

Healthy emotions are needed for children for wholesome personality development. But care must be taken to learn experiencing subtle emotions, and not always expressing emotions. Depending too much on expressive emotions leads to expectations and may cause disappointments. Many of the expressive emotions are artificial and sometimes commercial. We should neither get carried away with them nor get upset without them. That is the way to equanimity, peace, and real happiness

As the identities become stronger, emotions become more intense, causing harm to the body functions by releasing overwhelming and devious thoughts. They also result in a disruption in the outside world.

4. Memories:

It is the data collected as thoughts. When an action is required, thoughts are released. If only appropriate data is recorded, classified, and organized, and the rest of them deleted, the flow of thoughts is smooth. The actions that follow will be meaningful. But if unnecessary information is accumulated in the data bank, it will be very disorganized. It leads to uncalled for thoughts overflowing into the mind, causing confusion and overwhelming the system, which is termed as 'STRESS.'

The deletion of thoughts is not an active process. Just a command to delete will not work. The mind deletes unused information. By not repeating the thought or action related to that thought and not reinforcing the thought by emotions, the information gets deleted. When we notice strong emotions are emanating from certain thoughts, we have to wait for the emotions to settle down and later lighten the emotions by trivializing them by suggestions like it's ok, it doesn't matter, it's not important, etc.

Let me tell you a story about my friend and his wife to illustrate this concept better.

Manohar, a regional manager in an insurance company, one day dropped into my cabin along with his wife. They both looked visibly distressed and had tears in their eyes. Before I could even begin to ask them, what was the matter, the wife announced that she wants to divorce her husband.

Now, theirs was a three-decade marriage with kids married and well-settled. I looked at the husband. He complained, "See, doctor, I will be retiring from my service by next year. I got transferred to a far-off place. If I continue this year, I will have a lot of cumulative benefits after my retirement. If I take voluntary retirement now, I will lose all those perks."

The wife immediately chimed in, "Always money, profits, and benefits. Throughout his career, I have taken care of children and all the other responsibilities which he should have handled. Now I want to relax, and explore places with him, meet friends and relatives." He interrupted, "Just one more year, after that, we will have plenty of time."

She fired her last weapon, "I think someone must be there. Let him stay with her only, that's why I am asking for a divorce," she started sobbing. He was helpless to defend against the silly allegation. He was getting ready to hit back. I noticed that it was going nowhere.

At that moment, I knew logic would not work. I asked my friend to keep quiet.

I told him, "She is right. Why don't you take voluntary retirement? Is money the only thing in life?"

He was shocked. He thought I would be able to convince her with my logic. She was encouraged by my support and started to relax a bit. I started advising him, "Tomorrow itself, you resign. After all, how many years are left in your life, 30 more years? Yes, I can understand you have to pay back your housing and personal loans, and you will not receive your pension. What is the big deal? You don't require a big house in the heart of the city. You can sell it and move to the suburbs. A small dwelling for two of you will do, no?"

I could see the color of her face changing.

"To be honest, I was always a little jealous of your beautiful house in such a nice locality. If you are planning to sell your mansion, please keep me in mind," I added.

Next minute she bounced back, "No, Doctor, I didn't mean all that. I have sacrificed so much all these years. It's OK, just one more year, and I'll manage. He never asks my opinion for anything and takes me for granted. That's why all these problems. Anyway, let him do whatever he wants." She finished.

With it all sorted, everyone was happy.

"Logic doesn't work with emotions, tact does," Resource added.

Have you ever wondered why you're so forgetful when you are tense? It is because there are too many tabs open in your mind. With multiple thoughts and emotions, the mind is confused and unable to organize the memories. When you're working on a project and start worrying about your parents' health, you can do neither of them justice.

Multi-tasking, when done in a planned manner, is useful. But when it's done in a hurry, it will result in a poor product filled with mistakes, and then you have to invest more time in fixing it. It is like driving rashly on a crowded road trying to reach your destination quickly. It results in more delays due to an accident or traffic violation or an argument. Intelligent driving is the key. So, it is with life. Calm and planned thoughts with breaks in between will ensure better processing and, thereby, a stress-free life.

Memory is the data bank of thoughts, both short and long term; crude and subtle; obvious and hidden. The mind releases thoughts or commands, which is the basis of every minute of our life.

"One thing I love about memory is, it erases all the bad I have done to others, but remembers the harm others have done to me," I said. "The vice-versa is also true," added Resource, trying to make the topic easy, "I suppose that is the work of the ego." Yes, it's ego, and it is limited to the idea of me.

AS ARE YOUR THOUGHTS, SO IS YOUR LIFE

Every minute of our individual life is nothing but our thoughts, released from the data bank called memory.

The other day during my morning walk, I met two people who were acquaintances. The first one was wearing a Rolex watch, a gold chain, and rings, and was carrying a small bag of carrots. When I greeted him, good morning, he started complaining about the expensive vegetables and told me that He purchased only half the quantity of what his wife had asked for. The second individual, a lower-middle-class person, was also carrying a bagful of carrots as desired by his wife but with no complaints. He was aware of the expense, too.

I wondered who is rich in these two? The richness is in mind and not in the possessions. A person who is trained in combat shies away during a war, while the other, untrained, join the combat. Who is brave?

Bravery is in the mind, not in the muscles. Usefulness is not in our ability. Rather it is in our availability.

What our mind tells us by releasing thoughts is what we are, and that is what we do. So, collection, organization, and release of relevant data is the key to a smooth life. This data, when it identifies with "me" as self, emotions are created. When emotions overwhelm the system, innate intelligence is disturbed, causing diseases. Depending on the type of emotional disturbances, different body systems will be affected, and a variety of diseases arise. All these processes are not exclusive but are interdependent.

This is on a very superficial level, but to implement it, you need deeper knowledge. At the level of thoughts, stress is defined differently. The experience of everyone's life is nothing but their thoughts. The mind releases about 10 to 12 thoughts per minute for most of the people, whether they want it or not. That is its nature. But what exactly is a thought, and what's its purpose?

A thought is a command released from the accumulated data saved as a memory.

Thoughts are meant for action.

You can't create action without a thought.

The action may be physical, mental, or intellectual, but there is always a thought behind every action.

Thoughts are very subtle but powerful energies.

Thoughts create inventions, ideas, masterpieces of art, poetry, books.

Thoughts can create wars, extremism, suicides, and homicide. Human activity is ultimately an expression of collective thoughts.

If we get one thought for one action, the activity is then a smooth process.

But we have developed the habit of releasing at least ten thoughts for a simple need. You want to buy a pen for your day to day use. You go to a shop to buy it. You check the price, check the quality of writing, and just buy it. But you have started releasing ten more thoughts like I don't like the color of the cap, is it slightly costlier? I should bargain, so on and so forth. In the end, you are upset that the color of the cap was not green but blue.

When more than the required number of thoughts are released, then intellect will come into play. It analyses and filters extra thoughts and keeps them aside.

Here is an example to help you understand. Every day at 5 pm in your office, your unit head walks in and asks what you have done for the day. Before you answer, he starts shouting at you. You try to show him what work you have completed, and yet he threatens you with a pink slip and walks out. You can't even stand up for yourself.

So, every day when you hear the footsteps of the unit head,

your face becomes red, pulse rate goes up, and sweat props up on your forehead. You start getting a headache and go to your doctor, who promptly diagnoses it as hypertension with BP 150/ 100. You blame your unit head and your company as the cause of your hypertension.

You must know that all these illnesses have happened inside your body because of the chemicals released by your system. Nobody has introduced them from outside. It is your thoughts in response to a situation that is responsible. Situations, no doubt, are not in your hands, but the response by your emotional thoughts is purely yours.

Yes, it is happening without your knowledge because your mind is tuned that way.

So, you must relearn the process of thought generation. This will make you immune to external influences.

Your boss's outbursts are only the data you have received. You must have the know-how to delete/analyze and download options.

Similarly, with viruses of greed and fear contaminating your system, you must have a good antivirus called intellect. If you attempt to understand the reasons behind your boss's anger, you can see two reasons. The first, probably the correct one, is that he is just transferring his stress to others. In that case, you sympathize with him and choose the delete option. The other reason is maybe he wants you to quit the job and go, so he is putting pressure on you. Then you have to be careful and take proper precautions or make alternate plans.

Those thoughts generated and kept aside are energies with the need to act. They act on our different tissues producing small changes in the beginning. Similar repeatedly accumulated thoughts over some time sow the seed for the disease. Under favorable conditions, it sprouts into a plant. At this stage, the plant of the disease can still be plucked out like a weed. As it becomes a full-fledged tree, it becomes more difficult.

So, if there is the only release of the required number of thoughts, then the need for filtering by our intellect is minimal. The flow of life is smooth. The thoughts when they get attached to single unit entities like I, he, you, or narrower denominations like family, religious groups, friends, and foes, the life processes get more complicated. The friction that results from these causes damage to health.

"Then what is the need for the intellect?" Resource asked.

Intellect has three roles: one as an antivirus, for the data sent from outside. It helps you filter out fake news received through WhatsApp forwards. The second function of the intellect is to analyze the thoughts released before taking any action. The third role is for contemplating on complex issues, and for the mind to compile, classify, and conclude on dilemmas and controversies. This helps the mind to be calm and composed at all times.

Your intellect uses a tool called 'Why' to help you decide on matters and take action. For instance, you are offered a new job, or you want to start a new venture, or you want to take retirement; then, the first question you have to ask yourself is, why do I want to do this? You'll get an answer, then keep questioning the answers, too. Finally, you'll be in a place where you are completely comfortable and motivated to do that action. Then you can go about how, what, when, etc. of that action.

To my mind, the main role of intellect is for higher dilemmas and doubts. As you see, right now, we are using the intellect for analyzing and understanding the process of life and its ramifications. Similarly, we can use our intellect for contemplating concepts like death, the meaning of relationships, the universe, cosmos, etc.

But unfortunately, we have started using it for trivial things, like making smart decisions to get better deals, to win in a competition, getting awards, circumventing laws, etc. Overuse of intellect is like driving a vehicle, while continuously pressing the accelerator and using brakes frequently without reducing speed. The vehicle will wear out, be prone to accidents, and become dangerous for others on the road. But if you accelerate as per the road and traffic conditions and use brakes sparingly, the driver, car, and everybody is safe. I like to think of us as drivers. The life journey is akin to driving a car. The thoughts are the accelerator; intellect is the gear and brakes. If you use the accelerator depending on the road conditions, without changing the gears and brakes frequently, then the journey remains smooth.

As we were wrapping up, I noticed Resource jotting down the notes and preparing to leave. Before he left, he typically asked, "Where did you get all this knowledge from?"

TRIP DOWN MEMORY LANE

Resource left, and I, on my way back home, went back in time. The first thought process was set when I was in my final year of medical school. Just before the final year examination, I went to a temple to pray to God to get the best rank in my exams. I saw a small gathering waiting for a Swamiji to give a discourse. I joined that group to listen to some stories from epics for relaxation. A confident person walked in orange robes with a flowing beard and a smile on his face. He was Swami Chinmayananda, conducting Geeta Gnyana Yagnya. There was a simple question - What is religion? He explained it in a much simpler phrase - *'a way of life.'*

In those 10 days of discourse, he explained the relationship between body, mind, and intellect and its functions.

The whole extract of *Bhagavad Gita*, the song of the divine, is that you have all the rights to your actions but not to the results. Do it without any expectations. It worked wonders in my oral exams, where I always used to fumble. Then when professional and family responsibilities started, the philosophy of doing it with passion but without expectations was not working out for me.

We are all taught to assess and analyze the benefits we get before starting any work. What am I getting by doing this? This question is always on our minds. Supposing you have finished your engineering course and are searching for a job. You get a job offer. The first thing you look at is what the package is? If the package is tempting, you don't mind sacrificing your values, job satisfaction, family life, in turn sacrificing your health.

Then came an encounter with karma philosophy - what you do, you get it back, whether you want it or not, which helps in answering unanswerable questions. Whatever are the intentions of your actions, you get it back, both good and bad. I had put this simple theory on trial, and the results were quite convincing.

One incident baffled me in the early days of my practice. A close friend of mine who was a gynecologist by profession suddenly developed an autoimmune disease-causing weakness of limbs and threatening her routine life as well as her career. She was a disciplinarian, physical fitness freak, nutrition-conscious, multi-talented, multitasking, and lively. She was being treated by her neurologist friend. She was getting recurrent attacks for almost 10 years. But with sheer perseverance, faith, and grit, she could overcome it but unfortunately lost her neurologist friend to cancer.

If doctors, with all their background medical knowledge-are victims of diseases then what is health?

What is the source of all these?

Is there a way out?

Is our medical knowledge very superficial?

Is our knowledge only disease-centric?

Are we trained only for the treatment of the disease?

Is our understanding of life processes very shallow?

Is it our ignorance or arrogance coming in our way?

As I started introspecting about my profession, I found some interesting observations:

Doctors are products of the society they live in, and so represent the whole spectrum of society.

There are varieties of doctors who fall into these following categories.

Purely professional and technical: knowledgeable but not pragmatic.

Purely business like calculative, courteous, organized, opportunistic, profit-oriented.

Academic: teaching, research, publishing, training.

Entrepreneurial: establishments, innovative administrators.
Political: elections, posts, power-mongering, leadership.
Humane: patient-oriented, helpful, and empathetic.

Furthermore, knowledge started pouring in from different books on philosophy, Upanishads, gifted by my patients and friends. Gradually it started crystallizing, and I started counseling people on the concepts of I, the purpose of life, etc. And I saw people reversing many of the lifestyle diseases, addictions, dilemmas and confusion, anxiety, and depression, etc. And as I started explaining, my questions started increasing, my quest started expanding, and meditative processes helped me develop my knowledge. But the theoretical knowledge we acquire from books, attending classes, and analyzing the incidents are to be tried and tested at home, workplace, and the world at large. These processes are painful in the beginning because the established ideas and ways of thinking are to be demolished. In this path, what you encounter as obstacles and whom you consider as opponents, are the real gurus pushing you up to higher wisdom.

I started experimenting with my weaknesses, assumptions, and started practicing before preaching.

For Example:

Stopping all sorts of sweets for a month before advising diabetic patients to do so.

Fasting the whole day to advise obese patients to control their diet etc.

Walking barefoot on the streets to experience the real feeling of the earth.

I started freeing from the mold I had created around myself. So, my knowledge is partly accumulated and analyzed, somewhat intuitive, and synthesized knowledge.

I learned that there is no new knowledge to be developed. The abundant and complete knowledge is dispersed uniformly in the universe. Searching, downloading, interpreting, and application is our choice.

Rapid-fire:

Resource came the next week, thrust his chest forward, and lifted his hands up and pronounced – "Shoot!"

I laughed as I remembered our childhood game after each session. I made my hand like a pistol and shot questions at him based on the discussion held last week.

1. What is health?
"An expression of life."

2. What is disease?
"Imbalance in life processes."

3. What are the life processes?
"Four – Physical, Chemical, Energy, and Intelligence."

4. What is a living being?
"A physicochemical process that is driven by energy which is guided by intelligence."

SAGE 2
WHY HEALTH?

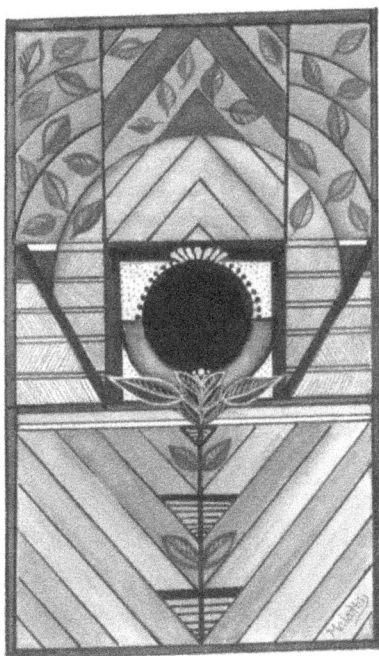

Resource was impatient through this whole process. He was keener on learning about curing diseases as opposed to understanding health. "Hey, Source, everyone has to survive and earn a living. They must build a career and settle down in life. We are bound to neglect our wellness, and why is health so important, anyway? I am a member of many health-clubs, as I try to take care of it but no avail," he said.

Listening to him, I realized that health is never posed as a question to a doctor by anyone because people have already accepted the fact that health is going to be affected thanks to the daily grind.

It also comes last on our priorities because we think we don't have the luxury to rest and think about it even.

I told Resource, "Health is the last priority for all of us. It comes after we have taken care of our jobs, entertained ourselves, and taken care of familial obligations.

We think that getting ourselves tested once a year and buying a premium health insurance is taking care of ourselves. Also, our priorities are so misplaced.

I have seen patients with reams of reports, but they won't act to change habits that harm them. Doctors keep prescribing medicines mechanically without looking at the problem holistically. What's more, I have met a patient who was 130 Kg, and worried about hair loss and not his obesity."

"Well, we learn the importance of health when we're afflicted with a disease or when there is a virus around the corner," Resource pointed out.

That's when I began to ponder. In our zeal to reach the top, all of us were eagerly trying to climb the ladder of success without noticing and maintaining the strength and stability of the ladder itself.

I asked Resource, "What is the single most important thing for success in any sphere of life?" Being the management expert in an MNC, he confidently answered, "It depends, in any profession – your focus.

In business – your acumen. In entrepreneurship – your attitude. For industrialists – vision. For a country – unity. For religion – discipline..." he was going on.

I interrupted him, "Stop, for all the things you're listing, health is the prerequisite. If we have health, we can achieve all of it easily and enjoy it too."

Consider This:

Can a doctor focus on his work if he is suffering?

What is the use of insight for a business person, if he's sick?

Where is the vision, if your vision is severely affected by diabetes?

The most united country, though by force, can be shaken by a strain of the virus and shut down.

What use is of religious discipline if you are bedridden?

If you are healthy, only then, any of these can be attained, accomplished, or even attempted. Even if you get all these easily and your health is poor, then it will all fall apart. With all these truisms dominating our conversation, Resource seemed to be getting bored.

So, we decided to sip some coffee and let our minds slip into contemplating on health.

I was reminded of one of my patients. He was the son of a wealthy businessman, and he complained of nagging pain in the anus. He was expected to sit for hours at the shop, but he couldn't. He couldn't speak of his predicament, and his partners thought he was merely making excuses so that he doesn't have to work. This insensitive approach made him depressed and suicidal. I was referred to his case by a colleague. I fixed his condition with a minor surgical procedure and counselled him, too.

I narrated this incident to Resource. I also gave him statistics for evidence that today the middle-income and lower-income groups are almost destitute due to health problems and treatment. It is a vicious cycle.

People neglect health to make money, and they end up spending more money to treat the diseases they have accumulated.

In the meantime, when they are ill, their productivity declines, which means lesser income and more stress. Their conditions make it impossible for them to work harder, and can't afford the treatment if they don't.

Furthermore, serious illness increases expenditure, affects relationships, and derails careers. Dreams are shattered, and accomplishing them gets more demanding. That's why they say health is wealth.

"Napoleon Bonaparte and Alexander the great could not accomplish their quest to conquer the world due to illness." Resource quipped. "So, the moral of the story is – health is the base on which anything can be created," he concluded.

Resource then asked, "If all these diseases are because of stress, can they be reversed? Can we get rid of stress itself? Every year we have stress management courses conducted by management and spiritual gurus of international repute. I have attended all of them diligently. After some time, they don't work. I am more stressed by these stress-busting courses than a regular office day. Do you have any tricks up your sleeve?"

Stress is not only the cause of almost all long-term diseases but also the reason for most of the problems the world is facing, including wars, terrorism, addictions, etc. So, a stress-free life is not an option anymore but a necessity.

"There are three ways of dealing with stress. But before that, I would like to know from you what stress is?" I asked. "Stress is that nagging feeling which will not allow me to have a sound sleep, and then everything starts irritating me," Resource responded.

I then asked, "OK! What do you think is the reason for stress?"

Resource said, "Stress is part and parcel of modern-day life. I just wanted to know what sort of yoga or meditation you practice to be calm."

I started by saying, "I want you to remove certain concepts from your mind."

1. Stress is not part and parcel of life.

2. Stress can't be or should not be managed. It is not even a necessary evil. It is a monster created by you, inside your mind, and you are playing to its tunes.

He interrupted again, "But the problem is with these people. Daily, I pray and do yoga. But by the time I finish my work, the boss is shouting at everyone, and the junior employees not understanding a thing gets to me. And, I am back to square one."

I told him, "Why don't you change your company?"

He replied, "Previous company was much worse. The boss was a dud. The salary was a pittance. They expected miracles from me. All these guys are the same."

I said, "You are right. You can't go on changing your boss, company, wife, or children. The whole world won't change for your sake." What you can do is change yourself. When you change, the world around you changes as well. Let me give you a simple formula to help you understand.

Stress = Expectations - Reality

For example, you have an expectation of one million rupees as your income. But you are getting only 900,000. The remaining is your stress. You can try to improve your income, but it's not entirely in your hands. What you expect is in your hands, though.

The other day, I was in my OPD, seeing patients. A couple came with a box of sweets, offering them to everyone to celebrate their son's passing in exams. "He got 38%. We were sure he would fail these exams, but he passed," they said.

After a while, another couple came with frustration on their faces and wanted their blood pressure checked. As the nurse was doing the needful, I inquired what the matter was. Together they announced that their son had done unsatisfactorily in exams by securing only 96%. "What is the use, Doctor? We sent him to the best coaching center, and he is useless. It's all our fate. We were expecting at least 99%," they said.

I counseled them by quoting the previous couple's example and asked them to support their son, who may be upset because he didn't fulfill his expectations.

We often see students dying by suicide after the results are announced. Farmers, entrepreneurs die by suicide every year in staggering numbers because they cannot repay loans that they've taken based on the expectations that their crop will yield, or they will make a profit.

Resource added, "I always wonder, how is that a politician

or an activist never dies by suicide? Despite repeated failures, they continue."

I explained, "Expectations can be managed in two ways. One has to think that there is nothing like a failure. I will go ahead, do what I have to, whatever is the result. If I cannot pay back the loan, I will go to jail, return, and start my life again but not end my life. Those who work for profits must think like this. The other thought process is, 'I am ready for failure.' 'I am fighting for a cause or an ideology.' So, dying by suicide defeats the purpose. 'I will fight until the end.' Those into politics think this way."

"Fine, I can manage my expectations. What about others' expectations of me?" Resource asked.

I answered, "Here's an example, your parents expect you to get 1st rank in your exams. You can only put your sincere efforts toward that goal."

Again, learn from the leaders: A president of a country can only do his best. No one can meet all the expectations of all his subjects. As I already mentioned, there are two approaches to deal with stress.

To dissipate the stress created in the day, through Yoga, meditation, psychotherapy, physical exercise, etc.

To suppress the stressful thoughts by medications like anxiolytics, antidepressants, etc.

Resource and Source were in a contemplative mood during their session; the phone rang, I disconnected, it rang again – 'the same number.' I picked up the call. It was one of my old patients, Lakshmi, sobbing, and narrating her plight. Resource was paying complete attention to what I spoke on the phone-

"Who? Manja? Your husband?? Oh! Party at a Dhaba. Hmmm. What happened? Loose stools? 20 times? OK, Saint's Hospital? Since how long? Four hours and waiting for an ICU? Blood culture reports? Oh, what does it say? You didn't wait, fought with them, and have transferred him to our hospital? OK. Is our staff not willing to admit him? Maybe because they see that the facilities are not enough at our hospital. OK, since you insist so much and are ready to accept any eventuality, I have no choice now. I will ask my staff to admit him. OK, wait. I am

getting a call from the hospital." She cut the call by saying that she is going home to arrange for the money. I called back to the hospital, and gave instructions to the nursing staff, "Start IV fluids, run the fluids rapidly, get investigations done. I will be there soon."

I left in a hurry, as Resource asked me to come back next week with an answer to what a disease is.

The next week, he came with a blueprint of 'building blocks of career.'

Rapid-fire:

Source – "It's time for me to shoot again. Hands up!"

1. Why is health important?
   "Health is the foundation of all careers."

2. What is the most critical thing for success?
   "Health!"

3. What is the factor that brings down our economic status?
   "Ill health."

SAGE 3
HOW TO BE HEALTHY?
HOW DOES A
DISEASE OCCUR?

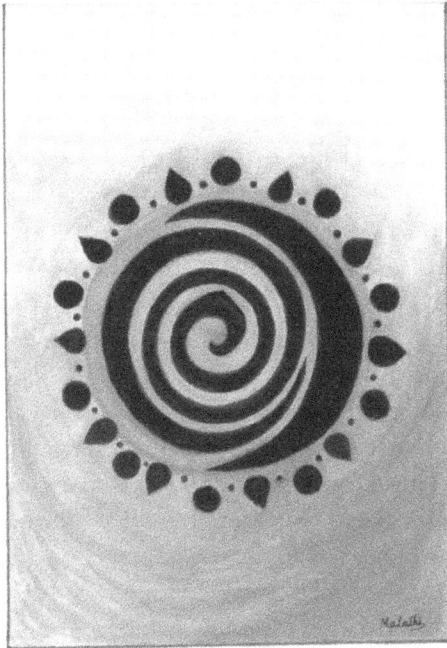

When Resource asked me, "How to be healthy and how does disease occur?" I found the question difficult to answer, despite my medical background. I could always quote the definitions I had learned from textbooks. I resisted the temptation to do that because that is information anybody can read off the internet and add to already prevalent anxiety.

I had arrived earlier than him this week for our little meeting. He came and announced, "I know you are struggling to explain what is a disease. Since I have first-hand knowledge of it, I will explain."

1. Diseases are the causes of all human suffering.
2. To be healthy is to get rid of diseases.
3. If we become healthy, we can be happy.
4. All the diseases are caused by environmental factors like pollution, contaminated food, water, unhygienic conditions, etc.
5. If we have enough money, then we can be healthy.
6. Technology is the answer to all diseases – vaccines, masks, sanitizers, antibiotics, nutraceuticals, supplements, PPEs, etc.

He then looked at me, triumphantly. He was so sure of his answers.

I told Resource, "I will bust all these myths one by one. But first, let me clarify that the disease has a process. It starts as a biochemical change, and then it becomes functional — where symptoms like pain, discomfort cause us to suffer."

Furthermore, our suffering increases when we tend to identify ourselves through our diseases. We say that "I am diabetic or hypertensive," instead of saying that I have diabetes. When we formerly address ourselves, we become sad, frustrated, and believe that something is wrong with us. We go into a denial mode.

These reactions will lead to mental suffering, which compounds the existing physical distress. The suffering from the disease itself is minuscule compared to mental agony.

The disease is a measurable physical entity, whereas suffering is a state of mind. I then proceeded to bust the myths he had about diseases.

MYTHS ABOUT DISEASES AND HEALTH:

1. Diseases are the cause of our suffering.

Not really. Because as a human being, you are likely to experience illness at some point in life. You have no control over that. Your job is to seek treatment and recover from it. Either you can stress about it or just do the needful and minimize the damage. Most suffering is mental than physical and hence optional.

2. To be healthy is to get rid of diseases.

Health is the basis of our life, and diseases are only guests visiting on and off. You can't wish them away! You must learn how to respect them and treat them well, serve them medicines, and not to say, "see you again."

3. If we become healthy, we can be happy.

We can get happiness by being healthy. Joy is one manifestation of health, but it is not the goal. Inner happiness is what we are made of, and we have to identify with that to be healthy.

4. All the diseases are caused by environmental factors like pollution, contaminated food, water, unhygienic conditions, etc.

Not all diseases. Some have a genetic component to them, and some are lifestyle-related. Environmental factors do cause a significant amount of conditions, no doubt about that, but it's also crucial to remember that different people have different levels of immunity and coping mechanisms.

5. If we have enough money, then we can be healthy.

Sadly, no. Health cannot be bought. Diseases can be treated, though. More money and insurance only means that you will be spending exuberantly on tests and procedures. I've met people who spend lakhs of rupees for procedures in high-end hospitals. They also don't want to quit drinking because,

47

well, they have the money to treat liver cirrhosis. This approach is wrong because your goal is to be healthy irrespective of your bank balance. You owe it to yourself.

6. Technology saves us from diseases

Yes, it can attempt to. If it could solve all our problems, then there would be no cancer, and we'd have had a vaccine to Covid-19 almost immediately. Technology helps us fight diseases, it ensures minimally invasive surgical techniques, but it cannot cure all diseases. Even if it does, there will be newer illnesses with time.

COMPREHENDING THE CONCEPT OF A DISEASE

Disease is a disturbance in the ease with which our body functions. It interferes with the life processes that we discussed earlier. There have been epidemics in the past like the plague, influenza that have ravaged nations just like the COVID-19. We didn't have much control over these diseases, and they can be understood as natural disasters.

However, we also suffer from human-made conditions like addictions, mental health issues due to trauma and wars, illness because of chemical over usage, etc. Now, isn't this an effect of the overuse of technology? It most likely is.

Resource grew serious and ruminated, "Every problem has a solution, and the solution has its own problem."

He then asked, "What precautions can we take to prevent diseases?" My response to his question consisted of a monologue that made him impatient. Here's what I told him:

All living beings have the mechanisms to survive adverse conditions and propagate their species. These mechanisms are innate and are called instincts. A street dog knows what to eat and how much to eat, without knowing the science of nutrition. A monkey knows how to climb a tree and to jump from one branch to the other without having to learn Physics. A bird knows when and where to travel for its survival. It can travel thousands of miles and learns how to build a nest with available materials.

As I was going away on a tangent, Resource remarked, "Okay! I get it. How do we connect with our instincts again?"

"Fine, listen," I replied and continued explaining.

Our five senses of perception, ideally, act as sensors that aid us in living. Our understanding of smell, taste, touch, sight, and hearing helps us make decisions usually. However, they seem to be disrupted due to the information overload that we subject them to. Stress and fear also interfere with their ability to function correctly. Let me give you a list of examples of where we go wrong regarding our lifestyle patterns.

1. We eat all three meals a day, irrespective of feeling hungry or not. It's an unwritten rule.

2. The quantity of the food we consume is based on our likes and dislikes instead of the need.

3. Quality or variety is decided by our accumulated knowledge. For example, vitamins, minerals, carbs, proteins, fiber, nutrients, and supplements are dependent on what our feelings tell us. At times, we feel like eating bread/ rice and less of proteins, or we crave fruits or pickles, which are indicated by the needs of one's internal system, but we overrule them by believing that something is good /bad, hot/cold, etc.

4. These days, people need to be told what to eat, how much to eat, and what position to sleep in. We complicate our necessary activities by trying to approach it scientifically or technically.

As mentioned above, the examples show that we have interfered with our instincts by trying numerous methods every day. It's crucial to reduce this chatter and let them do their work.

Forget about what is good or bad in the food we eat and its nutritional values, healthy and unhealthy foods, etc. All eatables have something useful for the body, and excess of any of these is harmful. Just don't pick one fruit or vegetable and eat only that because a blog post on the internet tells you it's a superfood.

Eat when hungry, stop when full, and skip a meal when you have already overeaten.

Here are some myths that I would like to debunk for you:

Myth: Eat breakfast like a king, because the body needs a lot of energy for your whole day's work.

Experiment: Skip breakfast and see. I had stopped eating breakfast for months, and nothing happened. I would eat lunch between 2:00-3:00 PM and still function well physically and mentally.

Myth: For better digestion, eat small but more than three meals a day.

Experiment: Have one meal a day and see what happens. Try the concept of intermittent fasting.

Myth: Your diet must be balanced and needs to include carbs, proteins, fiber, etc.

Experiment: Listen to your cravings and eat what you feel like, from pickles and dal chawal to a sprout salad. Eat local and seasonal fruits. Think about the early humans who were hunters and gatherers. They ate what grew around them, listening to their instincts.

Myth: Fasting causes weakness and diseases.

Experiment: Fast once in a while, to learn what hunger is and teach the systems to re-learn the mechanisms to shift to different metabolic processes.

Also, here's a tip, experiment with your exercise and sleep too.

Then gradually, you will develop your innate mechanisms to deal with different challenges in life.

Each human being is a different animal with its metabolism, characteristics, and behavioral patterns. So you can develop your methods of eating, sleeping, working, resting, etc., provided you don't depend on authorities in these subjects. You are your authority.

What is right for me may not be suitable for you. Despite

overwhelming statistical evidence from the most outstanding Universities in the world, you develop your own, follow, observe, and change as and when needed.

Every life is an individual, unique, and dynamic process.

"Alright, got it," said Resource. He then inquired, "Once you get a lifestyle disease, can it be reversed? Especially in the case of diabetes, because many people asked me not to treat it. Apparently, once it starts, there is no end; it only aggravates."

"I've heard this so many times from my patients," I said. "They finally visited me when it had progressed and told me that they thought it would go away or stay the same. They think that once they start the treatment, they have to continue it for life." Well, you can't wish a disease away. Here's what I have learned about diabetes through my experience.

CAN DIABETES BE REVERSED?

I have developed a different approach to diabetes, especially in regards to it being a lifestyle disease. My first-ever diabetes patient was a middle-aged, mid-level manager in a local factory. He had no family history of the disease. His body weight, BMI, blood pressure were all normal. He was physically active in his regular job, which was quite hectic, though. He was a vegetarian and hardly fond of sweets. His lipids were mildly abnormal. Usually a very cheerful person, he was looking dull and anxious. His blood sugar after the food was around 280 mg (normal <140). I started the treatment with the then available medicines.

However, I was unable to figure out why he developed diabetes in the first place. I discussed with physicians, attended diabetes conferences to understand the illness. This was the time when the IT industry was booming. Bangalore had become the IT capital of India. Soon, India had become the world capital of diabetes. Diabetology became the most sought-after specialty here, and all pharmaceutical companies started diabetic divisions or types 1, 2, 3, etc. Many multinational pharma companies invested billions of dollars in developing new molecules every year. Diabetic conferences sponsored by pharmaceutical companies were held every few months on a grand scale, with lavish dinners and cocktail parties to take care of hard-working doctors and help the needy patients who have diabetes. Fancy genetic theories on causes for Indians developing diabetes were propounded. Cytological and molecular level explanations were offered. There was a sea of new information, and something felt fishy because, to my mind, ignorance about the real cause of the sudden spurt in the disease was camouflaged by using intellectual words.

Alternative medicine wasn't far behind, either. There were big claims of curing diabetes through herbal medicine, Chinese medicine, and various diets. Despite all the latest treatment options, the progression of the disease hardly stopped. Complications were increasingly noticed, and the suffix 'pathy' was added to every organ to describe the difficulties. Neuropathy, nephropathy, retinopathy, to name a few, were some of the names coined, although the real meaning of these labels was not clear.

The patient was secondary when it came to deciding treatment options like whether to give them oral medicines or insulin. What was the wonder drug of this year was the source of all distressing side-effects the next. The hapless general practitioners and their patients were baffled by the surge of disease, complications, and treatment options. Neither mortality nor incidence was coming down. Although great minds were working on this illness, the thinking, however, remained inside the box.

As I started seeing more people with diabetes, I started questioning myself:

1. Thirty years ago, what was the incidence of diabetes? In a small town with a population of ten thousand, there used to be one or two diabetic patients, invariably heads of the family from the business communities. No one else had it within the same family. Very few people within the society, wasn't it?

2. Have Indian genes suddenly changed towards

diabetes? If so, how and why?
3. Indian anatomical figure with a big belly, is it new? And how many with obesity have diabetes?

Fortunately, I was one among the doctors who were not entirely convinced with the self-defeating theories of 'genetically prone for diabetes,' 'childhood malnutrition,' etc.

I started digging in. With every new patient, I started spending at least an hour to understand their daily routine, family, nature of work, relationships, expectations, etc. In the process, I started analyzing the fundamentals of glucose's role - its uses, supply, and disposal. I understood that whatever research is being done now is:

- To block the absorption of sugars from the intestines
- Increase glucose utilization by giving additional insulin
- Increasing production of insulin from pancreas by removing medicine
- Improving the functioning of insulin by reducing the peripheral resistance

There was also a new method to throw the glucose out in the urine. Then there was also the option of metabolic surgeries, where the doctor shortens the stomach and intestines.

The next best thing I could do was to talk to the patients.

Here's what I told them to explain the illness.

1. Sugar or glucose is almost the same for all practical purposes.
2. Sugar is essential for all living cells in our body, and a continuous supply of sugar is required, especially for the brain.
3. When we eat monocotyledons like rice, wheat, ragi, jowar, oats, millets, etc., they all get converted into

sugar in our intestines.

4. After that, sugar starts getting absorbed into the blood, and its level starts increasing.
5. Blood sugar needs to be kept approximately between 80 to 140 mg.
6. If it goes below 80, the cells start suffering. The more it falls, the more dangerous it is, you may feel faint.
7. If the sugar in the blood starts increasing above 140, the blood becomes syrupy. The more the sugar in the blood, the stickier it becomes. This means there is lesser flow, especially in the smaller vessels, causing all long-term complications.
8. Low sugars can cause immediate life-threatening complications. Moderately high levels cause long-term vascular complications like blocking blood flow in small blood vessels affecting the organs. Very high levels of blood sugar have different types of severe metabolic complications.
9. Because of this, the body has mechanisms to keep blood sugar level in that range between 80 and 140 mg.
10. When the sugar levels start rising after a meal, insulin is released by the pancreas into the blood to bring the sugar down to an average level by pushing it into the cells.

Now that you have understood how blood sugar levels and insulin work, let's get to the more confusing bit.

Imagine you're going for a walk in the morning on an empty stomach, and a dog begins to chase you. You run for your life, and your blood sugar levels drop to below 80. But, because your body also senses danger, other hormones at play are adrenaline, noradrenaline, and cortisol. These are called stress hormones. These hormones increase the blood sugar levels by using the sugar reserves in the organs.

Now, the same thing happens when dealing with a lot of emotions, say avarice and fear. Their mind is all over the place, and the body is sensing danger. All the stress hormones are activated. Sugar starts pouring into the blood from the reserves stored in the liver, muscles, kidneys, etc. But here, the sugar is not entirely utilized as there is no physical activity involved. As the blood sugar rises, the pancreas starts secreting insulin to bring the levels down.

If the mental stress continues, over time, the pancreas gets exhausted. It is an unfair fight between insulin on one side and so many other hormones on the other. Ultimately, the pancreas calls it quits. That's when diabetes mellitus Type 2 has officially arrived.

The doctors look at and debate blood sugar from different angles, fasting, after food, random, three month's average (HbA1C), etc.

They conclude that to decrease blood sugar:
    a.   Block the absorption from intestines
    b.   Stimulate the already strained pancreas to produce more insulin.

"This is like increasing income tax to increase the government revenues when the economy is in crisis, which will be counterproductive in the long run," Resource joked.

I added, "Or, increasing the sugar's excretion in urine and similar other ingenious methods."

Sure, these methods work wonders for some time, but the stress hormones are unrelenting. This fight against diabetes goes on with more innovation and experiments. The disease progresses with impunity, notwithstanding an array of oral medicines giving way to injections, pumps, artificial pancreas, and metabolic surgeries. Each method claims superiority over the other.

Meanwhile, the other effects of stress are taking a toll on the rest of the body and slowly and steadily damages the organs. Every specialist worth their name will come to the rescue of the patient. He will order a plethora of investigations and offer a more fanciful diagnosis and state of the art treatment. The patient will also be tempted to experiment with homeopathy and naturopathy, etc.

Resource commented wryly, "After all, this is a win-win

situation for all. Doctors, diagnostic centers, pharma companies, hospitals, surgeons, researchers, publishing companies, conferences, media, nutraceutical, yoga centers, special diet products, and whatnot. Rich patients are happy that they can afford the latest and most expensive tests, and medicines, while the poor curse their fate."

Resource then inquired, "Do you mean all these medical science advancements for diabetes, in particular, are wasteful?" I answered, "Not at all. They have certainly made a lot of difference in treatment and are indispensable. My grouse is that the enthusiasm and effort put in the treatment aspect of the disease should be in the prevention aspect. They should play a role, by way of educating the public about the reversibility and practicality of the processes to eliminate it."

"Don't you think nobody is interested in doing that?" Resource asked. "Maybe we are overreacting. Probably they were all burdened with the management of the diabetic epidemic and had no time to think differently. Anyway, I contend that the onus rests on us, as individuals, to take care of our health," I replied.

I recalled an incident of a young couple who were married for three years. They looked tense and came with a big file in their hands. They were diagnosed with primary infertility. They had visited one of the leading fertility specialists for the treatment. Last year they even tried ayurvedic medicine. This time they were advised in-vitro fertilization, the chances being good as all the investigations of both partners were within normal limits.

When I casually asked them how frequently they have intercourse, the husband triumphantly told me once every six months. He added that they either meet in Shanghai or Toronto, depending on their convenience. They had currently taken twenty days of leave to finish this project and go back to their respective countries where they are working.

They were tense as they had already spent one week just to decide what to do. They consulted me for an issue related to proctology for the lady; she took many supplements for her infertility. I explained to them that they only met once in a blue moon all these three years of married life, which caused her not to become pregnant.

When I checked their records, it was mentioned by the junior doctor but was somehow overlooked. I advised them to go out, have fun, without scientifically planning for pregnancy.

Life is not merely about working in high profile jobs. Life should be wholesome. After six months, she was pregnant and living together in Canada.

Too much dependence on internet information without using common sense and finding technological solutions for natural things causes newer issues. I want to conclude by saying that take it easy in life and you'll be able to prevent diseases.

Rapid-fire:

"Shoot!" Resource proclaimed.

1. Which authority do you follow to manage your health?

"You are your authority through instincts and intuitions."

2. Are lifestyle diseases reversible?

"Yes, through stress elimination."

3. What is the role of technology in health?

"Technology is for diseases; body sensors and common sense are for health."

DR. RAJASEKHAR RAMAKRISHNA MYSORE

SAGE 4
WHEN TO INTERFERE?

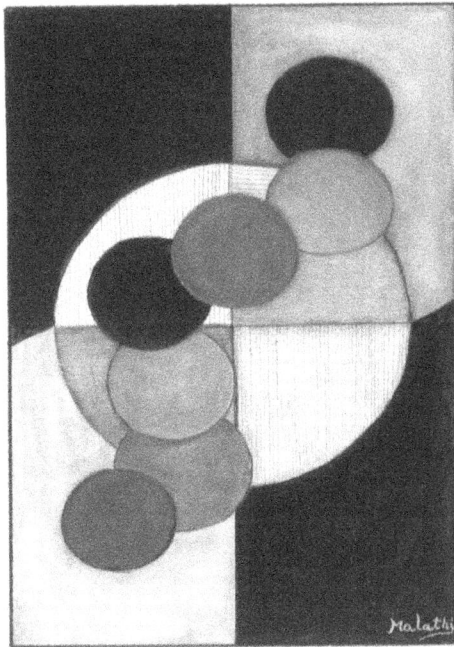

We often tend to put off treatment because it can be an unpleasant experience, or we have other priorities. This makes the situation even worse as it aggravates the disease. As we, Resource and I, began talking about the 'When' aspect of the disease, he came up with the following questions, "When should I start the treatment?

Can I wait till my daughter's exams are over? Or, can I wait till the launching of my work-related-project is done?"

These were some of the common questions that I often came across from my patients. I responded by reframing and classifying them as follows:

1. When to seek medical help?
2. When to start the treatment?
3. When to stop?
4. When to get a full health check-up done?

Here are the answers to these questions, so that going forward, managing your health becomes easy.

When to seek medical help?

Go by the following checklist to decide when to see a doctor and when not.

1. If you have minor symptoms like a headache because you went out when it was sunny and hot, try to get some sleep, and if it goes away, then don't see a doctor.
2. If you're dizzy because you're hungry, then eat and rest for a while. Watch such symptoms and see a doctor only if they are recurrent.
3. Seek medical advice even if you have a minor symptom like bleeding from an orifice, without a known cause.
4. Urgently seek medical help at the nearest hospital if the symptoms are severe, like unbearable pain, vomiting, diarrhea, and giddiness.
5. For chronic and lifestyle diseases – the importance of strengthening health, by way of yogic practices, primarily aimed at the system involved.

For example, Pranayama and breathing exercises for Asthma, Bronchitis, etc. Dietary modifications and exercises, games, sports, etc. for obesity, diabetes, lipid abnormalities, meditation, spiritual practices for stress-related issues.

When to start the treatment?

Before answering this, let me tell you what treatment means. It is the action to be taken when one is suffering or facing a disease. In the face of an ailment, you usually have four options.

    a. The first is action — you consult doctors and figure out what to do.

    b. The second is non-action — you plan what to do, read up about it, decide what to do, and not do much.

    c. Then there is the third, inaction — you just ignore the whole thing and try to wish it away, neglect.

    d. Finally, over action, it is more of a reaction, where you have anxiety about the disease. You are stressed and read up anything and everything about the condition, and catastrophize.

The first two methods are ideal and produce the best results. If you have been diagnosed with life-threatening diseases, then consult a doctor, make a treatment plan, and stick to it. If you don't know people in the medical community, then talk to a family physician and ask for recommendations.

Talk to friends and family for support. Reach out to experienced doctors for consultations.

As I was spouting truisms yet again, I noticed that Resource was looking at me with a blank expression. He was sweating profusely and looked pale. I immediately gave him an Aspirin, Sorbitrate, and Pantoprazole and called an ambulance. He was soon transferred to the Institute of Cardiology. In no time, my suspicions were confirmed. He was transferred to the Cath lab. The first five minutes were like an eon. There, I seemed to be in a daze, and there was a sense of Deja vu because all the cardiology cases I had presided over in my life flashed before my eyes. I signed the consent forms for Resource and waited for what felt like an eternity.

I was taken back in time when a 32-year-old software engineer came into my hospital with his pregnant wife. He complained of a burning sensation in the chest, and as we were going to get the ECG done, his pupils went up, and he collapsed on the floor. We tried CPR for 30 minutes, and then the person was no more. The wife was shocked and told us that he took an antacid syrup for the past six months for the burning sensation in the chest. The lack of seriousness and timely attention to the symptoms had cost the man his life.

Yet another cardiac case — a young lady who complained that I should have referred her husband to another hospital, when he was brought to my hospital in cardiac shock, instead of trying to resuscitate him.

The other mother blamed me for referring her daughter to a higher center instead of treating her at our hospital. Memories started rolling, pointing out how poor medical judgment can be while saving patients. But I also know that so many patients are getting well, some, despite our treatment. What if something goes wrong with Resource? I have no clue about his family or friends.

The past kept me busy in passing the time. Resource was soon brought out of the CCU after coronary angioplasty and declared stable. I was back from my reverie. I was finally processing what has just happened. I realized that I hadn't informed his wife and that we barely discussed our families.

Two weeks later, he recovered, and we were back in our discussions. His first question was, "You still haven't answered when do we stop the treatment?"

When to Stop?

The answer to Resource's question was, "Stop the treatment when the disease has been gotten rid of." He chuckled in response, "Or when the disease gets rid of us."

He then pointed out to me, "Don't you feel being a judge is the most cursed profession? They must judge and convict fellow beings based on evidence produced in courts. They are bound by the laws (or flaws) created by men, which will be changed or amended with time." Here's where I interrupted, "What of the profession where the investigator, judge, and the executor are the same person - — the doctor. Later the doctor is judged by the arguments on tv screens and unknown faces on Facebook."

We both knew that we were just moving away from the subject. So, we stopped at that.

"Hmmm. When to stop?"

I started recalling that I was entrusted with this responsibility. Whenever an older person is admitted to an ICU or needs ICU-care, the whole family has almost exhausted all their resources. They consult me concerning the next step.

One day my father went into a coma. I called my sisters and offered them two choices. As a doctor, I recommended he be shifted to a bigger hospital for higher investigations and life-support in the ICU.

And as a fellow human being, I told them, let's treat him here with minimum interventions; hope for the best and prepare for the worst with dignity. Fortunately, my father had confided in my elder sisters that he is against admission to more prominent hospitals and interventions. So, we followed his wish and accepted reality. To this, Resource responded, "Okay, your father was in a coma, not suffering in real terms. But what about those who have no desire to continue and suffer from minor ailments?"

I then narrated the story of Mr. Murthy, 97, a good friend of mine and a very pious and respected person. He came to me with a lot of swelling in both legs and water oozing from the skin (severe edema). In the past 25 years, he had undergone many surgeries in our hospital. This time he asked me, "What have I done? Why is He not taking me? All my responsibilities are over long back. I have no more desires."

This is one of the FAQs, by almost all senior citizens, who have had relatively good health for eight to nine decades and suddenly developed some trouble before their departure. My very active aunt asked the same question after being paralyzed, bedridden, and dependent on others for her survival. My simple answer is we don't allow Him to embrace us. We tie his hands with preventive cardiac, anti-hypertensive, and anti-diabetic medications, etc., take supplements and drips for strength, and by filling up all precious ICU beds. The guidelines I suggest below are my views as an individual, not as a doctor. They are neither mandatory nor advisory. They are only thought processes. I know that all decisions are to be taken by the individual affected, or by their attendants when the patient can't make his own decisions.

1. The decisions to continue or discontinue the treatment are to be taken by the person concerned, voluntarily and not out of frustration or extraneous factors like "I don't want to trouble my children," etc.

2. The decisions to be taken consciously, knowing all the possibilities. If one stops BP medications, then he may end up with paralysis and may become bedridden.

3. The decisions to stop treatment for any ailment should not be a temporary or an experimental measure. They have to accept the natural way of living without any interventions and continue all their activities — eating,

working, enjoying, etc., as usual.

4. Stop medications and add spiritual processes to improve the quality of remaining life.

5. Individuals must be aware that by making this sort of decision, they are not sacrificing anything or for the sake of anybody or society. For example, "I will not be a burden on society," etc. They are merely making a choice.

Resource then interjected, "But if somebody is on a ventilator for life support and is at the fag end of life, then?"

I replied, "age shouldn't be a factor on who gets to live and who doesn't."

• If the person is useful to at least himself when he recovers, he deserves a chance.

• If his illness's cause is reversible, life support like ICU, ventilators, dialysis, emergency angioplasty, etc., can be tried.

• However, if the cause of the illness is the aging process and there is irreversibility, and the consequences of recovery are worse than the peaceful end, then do we have the right to prolong their suffering just because we can afford it?

I could see the constant frown on his forehead slowly flattening, and Resource was looking more relaxed.

When To Get A Full Health Check-Up Done?

If a person is under a lot of stress at work and has an unhealthy lifestyle, they may require frequent checking of specific parameters. They may need to be persuaded to change their lifestyle rather than going for a check-up. Advantages of health check-up are: people with no apparent symptoms or those who don't care for their health, their abnormal findings may be picked up like high BP or high blood sugar. The disadvantage of health check-up is people with average biochemical values may think that their systems are robust. They tend to continue with smoking or alcohol or obesity only to end up with sudden life-threatening conditions.

On the other extreme, people with minor abnormalities develop anxiety neurosis or obsessive neurosis and make rounds of all hospitals. It's better to meet your family doctor often, get your general clinical examination done. Discuss with him the general and family issues so that he will be able to assess you as a whole with your medical and financial background guiding him. Merely getting an annual health check-up with hundreds of parameters checked at a discounted rate or arranged by your company may not be of much use.

On the other hand, a complete recording of history, followed by clinical examination and targeted investigations sequentially and follow up, will yield a better result than a blanket whole-body scanning/check-up.

Rapid-fire:

"Ready for firing??"

1. **When to interfere when diseased?**
   "At the earliest."
2. **Who should decide – when to start or stop treatment?**
   "The patient, after discussing all the pros and cons."
3. **What is the role of annual health check-ups?**
   "Decide after discussing with a family physician."

SAGE 5
WHO AM I?
AM I RESPONSIBLE FOR
MY HEALTH?

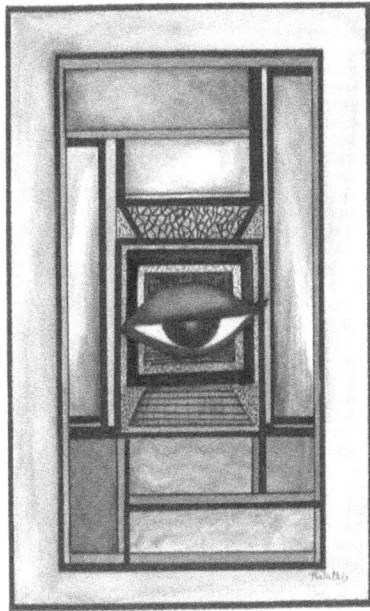

Since our last conversation was heavy, Resource and I decided to lighten it up a bit this time. This week's topic was all about getting to know the self. "Who am I?" I repeated the question and told Resource to recall the time he has asked me the same question. "Yes, you said something about me being the driver," Resource replied.

"Okay, let me ask you this, who are you?" To which Resource responded, "I am Raja, an IT professional. Son of someone…," he went on. I interjected, "You're not Raja. It is your name. If you change your name, will you change? You were there before you were named."

"Just like you existed before becoming an IT professional, and you'll remain even after you retire or quit the job," I added.

We are not just our bodies. They are merely hardware for our use. They change and are perishable. Your body is just a tool. You are what makes decisions and is composed of very subtle and powerful energy, which ensures the functioning of the body. This essentially means that you're the driver.

The energy that runs through your body, keeping you alive is a spark. It is a part of the cosmic energy and is eternal.

The main characteristics of this energy are happiness and peace.

This means that you, by default, are happy and at peace. However, happiness derived from your desires and actions is temporary. Happiness isn't your destination; rather, you are happiness. Being happy by gaining something and peace by getting rid of another thing is very temporary. Your identity is not with the hardware called body, mind, or intellect. It's with the internal, eternal, cosmic energy, made of happiness and peace. By changing from body-consciousness to energy-consciousness, you are relieved of many problems. The disease affects the body or its functions, not 'you.' It is imperative that you have a detached approach to disease. It must be technical and designed to fight the illness and must not become your identity. For instance, don't address yourself as a diabetic or a hypertensive person.

To explain this concept better, I have coined a term, 'INERGY,' it stands for intelligence-driven energy.

Inergy, when synced with your body, is a synergy that is the source of health. The root of disturbances in this synergy is the origin of the disease too. What I mean to say is that lack of inner peace causes illness. You must protect it to stay healthy.

As we were speaking about the sense of self, Resource had a realization of sorts. He told me that in a rush to climb the professional ladder, he forgot to marry. He joked that over time he found many lovers: SWEETY, BEAUTY, CUTY (Sugar, BP, cholesterol).

His next query was, "Who is responsible for my health or disease? I thought with regular annual medical check-ups, exercise, and diet, my responsibility was over, and whatever disease I am getting is my bad luck."

I replied, "When we are ill, we tend to believe that it is because of somebody or some situations."

How many times have we told ourselves that we are ill because we ate low-quality food? Or, because our children don't allow us to get adequate sleep? Or we tell ourselves that we have to work a lot and the office doesn't have a gym. We have blamed our spouses for causing us stress and called ourselves martyrs because we believe we sacrifice our time and health for the family and the organization.

You must know that health is inside you. It needs to be maintained by you through the optimum use of resources available. For example, if the food that gets cooked in your house has too many chilies in it and causes you acidity, you have a choice to modify it or dilute it while you eat. If your office does not have ergonomic furniture and affects your back, you have an option to modify it—request for a different chair.

If unhealthy working hours are causing you a lack of sleep, then you have the choice to adapt or quit.

If there's a pandemic, and you have no control over it, follow the norms advised at that point of time and accept that you are one among many.

If you are 'sacrificing' your health, wealth, or life, for someone or a cause or for society or religion or environment, then don't. 'Sacrifice' is the word to be used only for involuntary helpless animals – 'animal sacrifice' or 'child sacrifice.' Don't sacrifice yourself.

Now, coming to making decisions in regards to getting a treatment, choose wisely. Let me tell you two stories to make my point.

About eight or nine years ago, my cousin, Sudheer, called me while I was on a trip to the foothills of the Himalayas. "Hi Shekhar, my father had chest pain and was taken to a cardiologist. After angiography, he has advised a Bypass surgery. I will send all the reports; please advise me whether to get it done and where to get it done. You know, he is 86 years of age," he told me.

I thought it over, and once I returned and met my uncle, who refused the surgery after he was told that he could not ride a bike post-operation. He is fine now, and I even operated on him for an inguinal hernia. My point here is that the patients also have a right to decide for themselves. My uncle is doing well without the surgery.

So, who should decide about the health or treatment for the disease? It is the person affected, not anybody else, except in cases where the patient is not in a position to decide — in an unconscious state, in case of children, mentally affected individuals, etc. Even in those cases, what benefit the patient is getting should be the priority, rather than our affordability or availability.

The second story is of a relative who underwent a bypass just before he retired for a borderline blockage of vessels. He planned the surgery just before his service ended so that he could get a reimbursement. Despite the surgery, he has been living in pain exacerbated by post-operative scar for years.

Before we wrap up, there is a little bit I want to tell you about corporate health check-ups. There's a story again.

Guttedar from Raichur had gone to a tertiary care hospital for his routine health check-up. He had got all the possible tests done and also a whole-body CT scan with his political influence. He had brought his wife for some rectal issue, and she was posted for a minor procedure. At that time, he flaunted his thick grand file in a nice carry bag, and triumphantly declared that he is fit and healthy.

He booked her case for two days later but didn't turn up even after two months. She was brought to our hospital for the procedure much after the date. When enquired, his younger brother broke down and told that the very next day, Guttedar developed severe chest pain, and he was taken to the same corporate hospital, which declared him dead. The cause of death was an acute coronary syndrome.

When I noticed the discolored teeth, I asked him whether he chews tobacco. He accepted and mentioned that his brother used heavy doses of chewing tobacco, but never smoked.

He cursed the doctors that even after conducting all those tests, they could not prevent his brother's death. This fact, of chewing tobacco, was missing in his files, so no persuasion was made to stop it. I insisted that he stop chewing tobacco immediately before going for a battery of investigations, as suggested by the same hospital.

We must understand that there are different levels of health — individual, family, society, world, etc.

Individual health is your responsibility, and family health is a collective responsibility. Society's health is the government's responsibility, and world health is the World Health Organization's responsibility. The role of world bodies in health management is too vast and complex. National governments should allot sufficient annual budgets for health. The ministry of health should take a proactive role in necessary preventive health measures like sanitation, nutrition, awareness of healthy habits, fitness, mental and spiritual practices, potable drinking water, clean air, and vector control. Strengthening primary health care facilities, especially in rural areas.

As citizens, we must teach cleanliness both at home and in public spaces. Open defecation, urination, spitting, ill effects of smoking, alcohol, drugs, indulgence in food must be highlighted from childhood and discouraged socially. During calamities and epidemics, we must cooperate without selfishness. Remember, you are a part of the whole, and if everybody takes care of their parts, the whole will be naturally fine. We all try to correct the rest without first correcting ourselves. Only you are responsible for your health, and you can also contribute to others' health by being a role model.

Rapid-fire:

"Get. Set. Go!" Said Resource.

1. Who am I? Who are you?
"We are INERGY. Not the bodies."
2. What is your relationship with the body?
"I am not the body, but it is mine."
3. How are body and Inergy related?
"Body is Hardware. Inergy is Software."
4. Who is responsible for your health?
"I am responsible for my health."

SAGE 6
WHERE TO GO WHEN DISEASED?

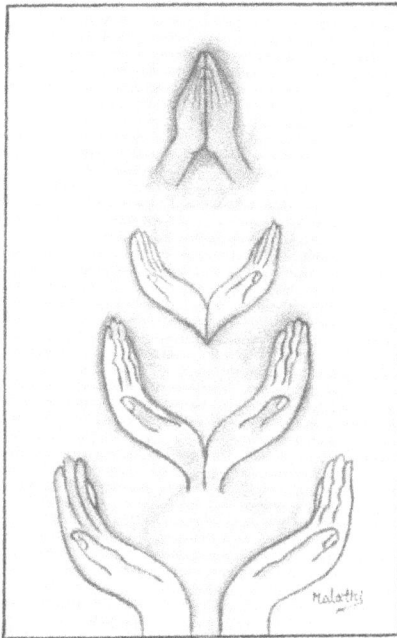

Let me tell you about Rukkamma, a lady in her 80s, who was diagnosed with inadequately controlled diabetes, hypertension, peripheral vascular disease, and other eye complications. I remember her very clearly as she was also the first patient of our nursing home.

Rukkamma would frequent the hospital for all sorts of diabetes-related complications. Her son-in-law *supported her, and surprisingly, though they were not well to do and belonged to a middle-class economic group, they never asked for any discounts on their hospital bill. Rukkamma had her cataract operated and had also gotten her leg amputated because of gangrene.*

Every time she came in, she would ask me, "Give me the injection they give in America to kill the patient," she used to tell me. However, I would make her understand every time that we had no right to take her life. But, after eight to ten years of constant struggle, we let her go peacefully without many interventions.

Every family has a 'doctor' in their home. Now, I don't mean someone with an MBBS degree. There is always a family member who is aware of the issues, takes an interest in the diagnosis, and keeps track of what the patient is going through.

Family physicians or general practitioners, or any doctor who is a good friend or relative who will have genuine concern and personal interest in the well-being of the patient. They are a significant player in private healthcare and are unfortunately dwindling nowadays due to too much dependence on high technology and super specialists. This is leading to many unsavory incidents.

I remember, Muniyappa in his 40s, was admitted with severe anemia (low blood counts). He had undergone investigations by super specialists like endoscopy, colonoscopy, CT scan of the abdomen, and was advised bone marrow biopsy. Knowing that he is a farmer who works day in and day out in fields, I ordered a simple stool examination, which revealed hookworms. I treated the worms; he got cured. So, the process of detailed history, clinical examination, and then higher investigations need to occur in this particular order and not the other way round.

When a particular disease or system is involved like heart, kidney, brain, etc., the specialist concerned is of real value. They have the requisite expertise and experience in their fields.

All the super-specialists will have more or less the same level of training and knowledge, so their approachability, their attitude play an equally important role in choosing them.

By now, I'm guessing you have an idea as to whom to consult and where to go when diseased. Still, while choosing a doctor, the thumb rule is this – Choose a humane doctor and not merely a technical doctor.

When I say humane, I mean to say that choose someone who considers you, the patient also a fellow human being and not a subject or a body to operate on. Analyze and select someone who can understand your religious beliefs, social and financial background, and are on the same page. This way, you will connect with the doctor, and this faith helps in your healing process.

Healing is at least 50% by empathy, if not more. Consider the doctor's experience and expertise than the kind of equipment used in the treatment. It is always better to choose stand-alone specialty units staffed by individual doctors than having new specialists visiting you every week, especially in cases of long-term diseases.

Follow the below-mentioned points while choosing your doctor.

- Assess his/her level of knowledge and ability to explain to you about your disease, treatment options, and its implications.
- Assess if you can connect to him personally and are comfortable with him/ her.
- See if the doctor is contactable in case of emergencies.
- See if he/she is patient enough to listen to you and clear all your confusions and dilemmas.
- The number of degrees, qualifications, places of consultation, the ambiance, discounts, Wi-Fi, insurance, other facilities like canteen and saloons are all secondary.
- To top that, the best reference would be someone who has been treated by this doctor previously.
- The doctor's passion for the subject and

compassion for the patient are the most important factors. A good rapport with the doctor is the basic requirement.

- The medical practitioner is not simply a qualified, trained medical professional, but also a friend, guide, well-wisher, and philosopher in your journey of health.

- Similarly, a patient is not merely a customer or consumer irrespective of whatever the law defines. He is a suffering fellow human being and is ready to offer his body to examine, cut, stitch, explore, and share all his emotions with the doctor, and not with anybody else.

- So, the relationship between a doctor and patient is unique and divine. It's a relationship of trust and affection.

- The best example I can quote from my experience for a doctor-patient relationship is between Mr. Nanjundayya and me.

Trust And Affection:

Nanjundayya was one of the first patients to get admitted complaining of asthma at our new hospital. In one of his multiple admissions, he was once brought gasping for breath. He was being resuscitated by mouth-to-mouth respiration and cardiac-massage by my doctor-wife, with the help of a maid when his breathing and heart had completely stopped. I was explaining the seriousness of his hopeless condition and preparing his wife for the inevitable. To our surprise, he suddenly took a deep sigh, thanks to the continued resuscitation. He completely recovered, only to be readmitted many times with recurrent asthma attacks and severe, unexplained pain in his leg. He was at least 20 years older than me. During each admission, I used to jovially accuse him of coming late to the hospital and testing my efficiency and proficiency at what I do. He, in turn, would accuse me of expecting him to get admitted with minor breathing problems so that I, as a doctor, could earn more.

Unknowingly, a special bond had been formed between Nanjundayya and me. He would always stir something up during his discharge and would not pay the entire amount. However, I would make fun of him and let him know that he would come back anyway, and we would get our money when he gets admitted the next time. I always wondered why he chose me. He would not go to any other hospital or doctor. He always came to me, and I was not even a lung specialist. I asked him this, and his reply meant the world to me. He said, "I don't care for all that, I only know that you are my well-wisher, and you'd do only the best for me."

However, during his last admission to the hospital, he was very sick, and he expressed his loss of interest in life. His last words were very moving. "Don't worry! Once I die, I will not abandon you. I will become a spirit and move around your hospital, protecting all your patients. You still have to serve many more people like me." – These words haunt me even today. It has been imprinted on my memory.

During our talks, I noticed Resource listening seriously for the first time, and I also saw tears rolling down his eyes for the first time. I did not ask him anything. After a few minutes of silence, he spoke up and told me that he had decided to stop using all social media accounts and minimize his internet usage for medical issues. Something did not feel right, and I corrected him, saying it was not the media at fault but us. If it is used in the right way, social media could be a boon to humankind. And as far as it goes for the use of the internet, today's communication and connectivity have no limit, thanks to the internet. Back in the days, the information about the latest developments in western countries in medicine used to take a decade to be implemented in India; however, at the moment, these latest techniques can be practiced in real-time, or even before them.

Role Of The Internet:

The internet is a great place to look for sources and references. That said, do not believe everything that pops up on the internet. Be sure to use your discretion before jumping into anything.

When it comes to medical usage, the internet can help us with the following things.

1. Apps to search – nearby doctors, specialists, facilities like lab, etc.
2. Maps to search locations
3. Websites of hospitals/doctors, to know details of facilities, contact information, and booking, etc.
4. Online consultations during the lockdown.

Refrain from googling your symptoms. Take it from me, most of it is incomplete and sometimes very misleading. For instance, searching for a simple headache symptom can show you results of brain tumors and other deadly diseases, and this might, in turn, affect your mental health. The stress you undergo after googling these symptoms will cause more problems than you can imagine. Let me tell you a story that emphasizes how wrong it is to seek the internet's help for your diagnosis.

Years ago, Pravin, a software engineer, visited me in an anxious state. He asked me to examine his neck. He told me he had cervical lymphadenopathy.

I asked him about the symptoms, and he said to me that he is aware that he has cervical lymphadenopathy and wants me to conduct tests. He spoke about swelling in the neck and repeatedly asked me to order more tests. He had an asexual encounter with an unknown person and read about AIDS.

Then he also showed me a thick file of reports from various reputed hospitals and test results. All the reports were normal, and yet the man was sure he was ill.

He had been advised to seek psychiatric help, but he hadn't done so. I told him nothing was wrong with him, prescribed an anxiolytic, and asked him to come for a counseling session after two weeks.

After I spoke to him, I learned that he had too much information through the internet, which was inducing paranoia and phobia. I talked to him and explained life, its processes, and health.

I taught him a thing or two about meditation. After three sessions, he was good to go. Two years later, he married and is now living a happy life.

Pravin, who was overloaded with information, suffered a lot for a non-existing disease because of it but fortunately reversed it at the right time with the right advice.

Where To Go When Diseased?

"Hey Source, before I forget, what happened to that Manja?" I asked, "Which Manja?". "Arey, that patient, who was shifted from Saint's Hospital to yours, that day when you left in a hurry..." he helped me recall. Let me fill you in on Manja. *On my way back that day, Dr. Ramya, who was a 'duty doctor' in our hospital a few years ago, called me, "Sir, Me, Dr. Ramya Patel. I completed my Emergency Medicine specialty, and I am a casualty in charge at Saint's Hospital. I am calling you because one patient, whose condition was terrible, got transferred to your hospital about an hour back. His blood counts are very high. He is in 'Septic Shock.' Please send him to a higher center immediately."*

I thanked her for the information and reached the hospital quickly. To my relief, Manja's bed was unoccupied. I thought he was already transferred to somewhere else.

But I saw him coming out of the toilet, with his trademark big smile, with almost all his teeth visible. He told me he does not remember how he reached the hospital and could not contact his wife. It was a simple case of severe dehydration due to loose motions leading to shock, revived by simple fluid replacement. After three days, it was Dr. Ramya Patel's call again, "Sir, that patient's friends, who were admitted along with him, one person expired, and the other is on dialysis, despite large doses of higher antibiotics. What happened to your patient?"

I told her about the dramatic recovery of Manja, who went back home the very next day. The high white blood cell count was probably due to severe dehydration, rather than infection. The usage of strong antibiotics in high doses might have precipitated renal failure in others.

Resource was listening intently with a gaping mouth. He asked me about the go-to place whenever there arises an issue. I replied, "Where to go depends on multiple factors — systems of medicine and level of the institutions, which depend on individual beliefs, preferences, and affordability."

Systems Of Medicine

I.   Medical institutions

1. Ayurveda
2. Homeopathy
3. Naturopathy
4. Allopathy (Modern medicine)

II. Palmist, Astrologer, Temple Priest, Prayers, Austerities

The systems of medicine, though look exclusive, in practice, the doctors themselves will be using different methods for their personal or family members. AYUSH doctors will be using more pain killers, antibiotics, modern medicine practitioners, and vice versa for their family members.

Each system of medicine has its advantages and disadvantages. Drugs derived from nature do not have side effects or are not harmful is a myth. If something affects, it will have some side effects; after all, it is some chemical ingredient, extracted or modified, which will be working on the chemical processes of the body.

Even simple water above the need can be harmful to those who have kidney and heart ailments. I remember one of my patients, who had no complaints what so ever in the anal region, had taken cleansing enema therapy, had lots of loose motions, and came with prolapsed piles, for which I had to perform surgery.

No single system of medicines is superior, and it is not the system, but the practitioner that makes the difference. Every practitioner knows the limitations and drawbacks of his plan, and if he advises accordingly, instead of bias or ego, it will be useful for the patient.

So, the system of medicines one chooses is to be guided by the following:

1. The patient's knowledge, experience, and faith.

2.   Diseases that can be lethal or dangerous and require immediate attention are treated by allopathy (modern medicine).

3.   Minor ailments and chronic diseases can be treated with other systems of medicine.

4.   Many symptoms with no known cause, also known as psychological or psychosomatic diseases, may respond to 'Miracle/Divine' interventions like prayer, austerities, and religious practices (provided there are no harmful effects). Though they are called the placebo effect, as long as the person is relieved, it should not matter.

Level Of The Institution

1.   Clinic – a single doctor
2.   Polyclinic – multiple doctors
3.   Small hospital – owned by doctor/doctors
4.   Large hospital – owned by doctors
5.   Stand-alone specialty hospital
6.   Corporate hospitals

Single Doctor Clinics
They are owned by qualified doctors – dwindling in numbers.

Advantages
Single point of care, accessible, affordable, individual attention, and the doctor is familiar with the patient and their family background.

Disadvantages
The doctor should regularly update his knowledge in all branches and be in touch with specialists for an opinion as and when required. When the doctor is on leave, it gets difficult to replace him/her. Trust and goodwill become the key factors here.

Polyclinics — Multiple Specialists In One Place:

Advantages
If any cross-referrals are needed, it will be easy and saves time. Many will have attached laboratories and diagnosis centers for convenience.

Disadvantages
Possibility of exploitation.

Small and Medium Hospitals — Owned By Doctors
All facilities for treating regular diseases – fever, gastroenteritis, injuries, and admissions, common surgeries can be done, with lesser cost and a single doctor in charge. Cost-effective.

Stand-alone Specialty Hospitals:
For the eye, ENT, Dermatology, Proctology, etc. usually surgical hospitals on a day-care basis. Simple processes, the treating surgeon, is accessible and involved from the first consultation to post-operative care.

Corporate Hospitals
They have a different module, very high investments, and are managed like companies with balance sheets, high-level marketing strategies, and concentrate move on, high return departments, and have 'Hire and Fire' policies for the 'Doctor.'

Advantages
High-end technology with very high investments is available for patients who can afford the luxury. You can also experience a professional approach and the 'wow' feeling, grand ambiance, cafeterias, parking spaces, etc.

Major accidents, emergencies, natural disasters – well equipped.

Disadvantages
They are super expensive, less personal approaches. More

commercial and less humane.

The Flow Chart:

Clinic/polyclinic → needs admission → small hospital, stand-alone specialty hospitals → Major illness, emergency → Larger hospital with ICU (mission hospitals, corporate hospitals, government hospitals).

Government Hospitals:

All are not up to date and appropriately staffed. Corruption, influence, negligence is all possible. There are some well-equipped specialty hospitals like cancer hospital, neuro/mental hospital, cardiac hospitals. They have qualified doctors as well. Affordable/free, but they are usually overcrowded and practically have no personal attention.

Personal factors that come into play while choosing the hospital

General Guidelines:

1. Affordability.
2. Personalized care is expected.
3. Approachability and contact ability to the concerned doctor – post-treatment.
4. Non-medical services are expected, like elegant rooms, food, TV, Wi-Fi, etc.

Let me tell you of another incident to stress on why choosing the right hospital and doctor matters. I remember one of my patients, a VP of an MNC, getting admitted to a corporate hospital's ICU for Gastroenteritis with mild dehydration. He had to undergo many investigations and had to deal with too many specialists pouncing on him. Sick of all this, he approached me and told me how uncomfortable he was at that corporate hospital.

However, I did not see anything wrong in the way they were

treating their patients. I mean, they are huge, and being at the level they are in, they have protocols and steps that they will have to abide by, irrespective of how trivial your disease is. I told him, "They have not invited you; you went there. They have protocols to follow and have less discretionary powers.

Their system works that way, and that is right for their level of medical care. For minor ailments, if you go, you have to accept all those." We have to understand that different medical institutions have different protocols and have to be intelligent enough to use it for our benefit. The system of health management in that particular country also plays a significant role. Some countries have well-established government-sponsored and controlled free health services. Here the financial burden for an individual is minimal, and the facilities available are equal.

But the individual can't choose the doctor or the hospital, the place, time, or even the treatment options. On the other hand, some countries have private medical care with medical insurance backing up finances. Naturally, insurance companies dictate the terms of treatment with their profits as their philosophy. Some other countries have a mixture of both. Government hospitals with necessary facilities mainly for the less privileged, whereas private institutions with or without medical insurance offer support for the affordable. Here the individual has the freedom to utilize the facilities according to his affordability and needs. A few countries have no policy on healthcare, and it is free for all kinds of options. It is mostly chaotic. So, every system has its pros and cons. The individual should choose based on his intellect and intuition, rather than fear and greed.

MEDICAL INSURANCE:

Resource gave a sermon: "Life insurance is a tricky business. It is no different than betting. You deposit a certain premium amount and bet on 'if I die.' The insurer bets on 'you won't' after ascertaining certain factors. If you win (die), somebody gets the benefit. If you lose (live), somebody else gets the service. So, as nobody usually wants to win this bet and it all works out in the benefit of the insurer."

I added: "In medical insurance, you pay a premium dictated by the insurer and bet on 'getting a disease' in his list. He bets on 'your health' after excluding pre-existing, likely acquiring diseases, and studying all your parameters and your past. Here if you win by getting an infection in his list, you have a limited choice of getting treated with 'conditions applied.' Here a third party is also involved in the actual service provider (hospital), and his hands are 'tied up' by the terms and conditions dictated at the time of their 'tie-up.'

Many who have taken the 'Mediclaim card' are unhappy because they have spent so much money for years and did not get an opportunity to encash it! On the other hand, others are excited to utilize the 'cashless' services from premium hospitals. They get back more than the premiums they would have paid!"

There was this permanent smile on Resource's face. Sitting next to me, holding my hand, he started talking about his personal life.

He told me about his father's health, and he was being transferred very often (repeated transfer to remote places and punishment postings are signs of integrity in government service). He told me that his father had started to lose weight but was stubborn about not taking 'English Medicines.' He was being administered homeopathy treatment from a primary school teacher.

However, when his situation worsened, he was rushed to a government hospital, but was declared 'brought dead.' He told me how his father's death brought about many hardships to him and his mother, with no 'unaccounted wealth' and only pension to take care of them.

Not wanting to burden me with his struggles, he cut short the story by telling me that his mother also joined her husband. In his quest to survive and prove himself, he forgot to marry and make a family. "I was happily unmarried, but don't be jealous," he said.

However, let me tell you about my three girlfriends — BP, Sugar, and Cholesterol at the same time.

"Can humor save a person's life, despite the problems in their lives?" I asked Resource. He was simply staring at me.

I narrated my story to him. After working for about a decade and returning from abroad, my wife and I started a small clinic. The first day, I got an SOS call from my cousin that my aunt had fallen from the cot and suffered an injury. I rushed to her house with a stethoscope on my shoulders. A stethoscope is like a gate-pass to crash any building with ease.

Resource interrupted me here to share one of his funny encounters. "Whenever I had to visit a big charitable hospital to see some of my colleagues at unearthly hours, I used to ask for my company doctor's help. He, with his white coat on his left shoulder, and I, with his stethoscope on my shoulders, would sneak through the side gate, where only doctors from that hospital were allowed. That time, I came to know why skin specialists and even psychiatrists carry stethoscopes as a matter of precaution. I also understood how a stethoscope on our shoulders makes us feel that we have descended from heaven. I am sure doctors will never abandon stethoscopes for any other fanciful gadget," he said.

To this, I replied, saying that the stethoscope had stood the test of time, at least as an ornament of aura! "For those who don't know, it is priceless, and some of them don't know how to use it," I added.

After this anecdote-sharing, I got back to narrating my aunt's story. When I rushed to her, she was in severe pain. Swallowing her pain, she chuckled and said, "As usual, I have managed to break one of my remaining bones that aren't fractured yet," and she challenged me to do a good job putting it back together. Typical Gopamma, my favorite aunt. Wondering why I am talking about my aunt now? Well, her story is not just about the fractures. It is about how she faced her life head-on. I'm sure you will learn a lot about life values as you get on with her story.

THE SAGA OF GOPAMMA

As I'm told by my father, he and his siblings were born to a low-income family where a second full meal on any day was a celebration. Gopamma was the eldest of the four siblings, and their father died when they were too young to remember anything. She was married off to a man from a wealthy family when she was about nine, hoping to get rid of one burden.

However, the family was not aware that Gopamma had been married off to a man who had already been married to another woman. He had left his first wife but wasn't divorced yet. Probably there were no laws restricting men from practicing polygamy back then [Pre-independence era].

The story unfolded further when the first wife, who was also my grandmother's sister, joined the family bandwagon, after a compromise with the real judge at home. I wondered how our hero used to manage his two wives and their kids living under a single roof. Probably that is the reason for having an open sky roof in the center of the building.

Each time I visited their house during my summer holidays, I used to see different situations. Gopamma and Nagamma were close buddies at times, trying to seek revenge on their hero. Other times, they would act like sworn enemies and attack him individually.

However, individual or collective, their efforts did not have any effect whatsoever on the hero. He never lost his composure or poise, always trying to play on his harmonium at night and attending the club in the evenings.

Unfortunately, he passed away in his 90s before I could collect the secret of his peaceful life. The Nobel prize for peace narrowly eluded him, I suppose!

In the meantime, Gopamma was managing her asthma by swallowing liberal doses of steroid pills at will. She did not notice her bones becoming brittle, thanks to the side effect of steroids. She also had to deal with other family issues like her children's health, their marriages, some of them going far away. She also had to witness the switch from a joint family to a nuclear family.

One thing I liked about Gopamma was that, even with so much happening, not once did I see her complain or whine about anything. There was hardly any bone which was not fractured in her body due to osteoporosis. All varieties of orthopedic implants could be spotted inside her. She always used to joke, saying that her body could be seen in a museum for bone doctors. I think she used humor as a way out of her pain.

However, the bone that she broke in her left arm could not be fixed due to technical issues, and ended up developing a false joint in the middle of her arm.

I visited her once just to check on her, and I found her knitting something. The wooden ball rolled away from her, and when she tried to stop it, her left arm bent at the false joint and went behind her torso.

She laughed loudly, and with the help of her right hand, slowly pushed it forward and continued her knitting. She announced that she was knitting a sweater for her granddaughter, arriving from the US next week. She was in her late 80s then, and this was her enthusiasm, despite all her hardships.

Whenever she had a fracture, I used to ask her whether I should inform her son; her reply was that he was a neurosurgeon and that he would not know anything about bones. "He will be worried. Leave him be. Let him serve the people. Whatever you can, do it. Otherwise, leave it," – this was her standard response.

She suffered another fracture, and when I asked her what had happened, she said, "Bones are there to get fractured. Otherwise, will my stomach get fractured?" Well, I had no comeback.

I don't have much idea about her educational background (not beyond 7th standard, I think). I doubt whether she had attended any spiritual classes. She was not reclusive and enjoyed every bit of life to the fullest, in her way. Each cup of coffee she drank had at least half a cup of sugar! When I saw a big rat running out of her kitchen, she said, "It's OK, they have a right to live!" This was the kind of positive attitude she had towards life.

Her secret was this. She was independent. She did not expect anything from anyone, having generously helped many. She did not expect anything from her children as well, who, by the way, was very well-to-do. She was straight forward, spoke her mind, but also made sure not to hurt anybody's feelings. She was a very broad-minded lady. Very liberal in her views, attitudes, and treatment towards others. She accepted things the way they were and made the best out of it. This was the motto of her life. She lived her life into her late 80s and was a living example of a karma yogi. I see her as my Guru. She outlived her problems and diseases, not with sheer grit and will but with a little wit and humor. So, answering the question raised earlier, yes, humor can save a person's life.

What Is The Moral Of The Story?

1. Misuse of medicines results in diseases. Gopamma's bones become brittle because of the misuse of steroids
2. Gopamma's identity was not with her body, but with her Inergy, which kept her happy till the end.

As I was narrating all this passionately, I saw Resource being all inattentive. I had lost him. He was sweating. He started muttering something. "Source...Sekhar...Sekh..." I heard Resource say. "Oh my god! Not again!" I muttered.

But I did not panic, I gave him a spoonful of sugar, and he came out of his hypoglycemia. "Haven't you eaten breakfast? Or have you taken more Insulin?" I asked. "Neither," he said. "In fact, for the past three days, my sugar levels are falling. I am reducing my insulin dosage. I am really happy!" he added.

"Wow! You are reversing your diabetes!" I exclaimed. He did not ask any questions. His face lit up. With a broad smile, he told me that he was looking for a lady to marry. 'Suicidal or homicidal,' I thought to myself. I wondered if there was anything like 'Diabetic cerebropathy' or some 'mento-pathy'?

Resource's blood sugar was within normal limits, cholesterol was almost normal, his weight started declining, and age started reversing. Finally, our Resource had discovered the real identity of life — the Inergy (Happiness energy) and was hooked onto it. He has regained his health.

He made one last prophecy. "Source, you will write a book on health," he said and smiled, "You know why? Whatever we have discussed now has helped me, and it needs to be recapitulated and revised once in a while so that the transformation should be continuous and complete. I don't want people to take these pearls of wisdom after the diseases hit them. We usually don't listen to suggestions when we are healthy. We take our good health for granted. We will only understand it's important when we are not fit anymore. A book will be handy, and people can go through it and help themselves." He thrust an envelope into my hand; thanked and walked away. I started asking myself, "a book?"

Why Does One Write A Book?

- When one thinks that one knows too much and nobody listens to them!
- When one has good language skills to attract people's attention and make a living out of it.
- When somebody ghost-writes and promises a fortune from it. I am not a celebrity!

Why Does One Read A Book?

- Time-pass. When one has nothing to do.
- To gain knowledge and learn about something that the other is an expert on.
- Fun or thrill, depending on age.

Why Do People Collect Books?

- Some are obsessed with buying, wrapping, and gifting books. They stack them.
- Some borrow books on a non-returnable basis and stock them.
- Many want the world to know that they are 'well-read.' So, they 'showcase' them.

I did not know whether he was making fun of me or praising me. Either way, I ignored and forgot about it.

Rapid-fire:

"Hey, transformed man, face the firing!"

1. **Which system of medicine is preferred?**
   "Depends on your faith, evidence, and situation."
2. **Which level of a medical facility?**
   "Better guided by a family physician."
3. **Which doctor?**
   "In the order of humane > expertise > experience."

SAGE 7
WHICH WAY FORWARD?

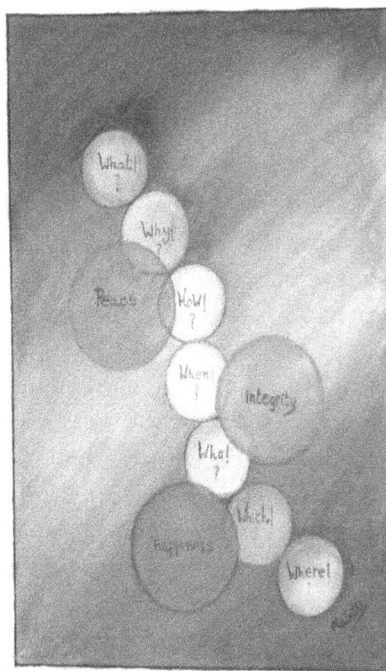

Days and days of discussion between Resource and I dragged me into more in-depth explorations of life mechanics. Health is not some status to be achieved. It is a dynamic process to be enjoyed throughout our life. We are all born with different levels of physical, physiological, mental capacities, and inclinations. So, we are all distinct, and let us start acting with that understanding.

Some of us have manufacturing defects (defects by birth) due to software errors or otherwise. They need to be supported, corrected and helped. All of us need to enhance our capabilities and improve our present abilities. This process is a lifelong effort.

We are all unique in physical, chemical, and mental makeup. The maintenance, further developments, and future updates are also unique to an individual's capacity and needs. No single method or mechanism will apply to all.

There is much advancement invented and developed in the outside world. To name a few, diet, nutritional supplements, energy boosters, dance, music, art, fitness exercises, yoga, meditation, religious rituals, prayers, spiritual practices, external cosmic influences, inner energy manipulations, etc. Each claim to be superior to the other.

All these are useful apps, but will they suit a group of individuals? We must have the capacity to develop the smartness to decide which, when, and how to use them. None of these give permanent solutions as the process of life itself is in constant flux.

Each person's journey is individual and modified by himself. There is no single right way or the only way to live. But there are guidelines on how not to live. The disturbances in the physical, chemical, energy, and intelligence processes of life, if identified early and action taken to modulate them, then the maintenance of health becomes a smooth process.

Signs Of Disturbances In Physical Processes:

Discomfort or uneasiness in the body parts is the earliest sign, followed by sensory irritations like itching, burning, and later different pain grades. If we identify and corrective action is taken at the earliest sign, physical health damage can't come to fruition. For example, though it looks brave and gives a feeling of achievement when a person tries to attend his work with the help of a cup of coffee and painkillers, after a tedious overnight journey with a lot of discomfort in the body and feeling exhausted. He will be damaging the body in the long run and later imagining or claiming that as a sacrifice is fooling himself. The best way is to plan properly to prevent this sort of issue or take appropriate action immediately. We are not here to take care of others at our cost. We are only a tiny part of the whole. The world moves on with or without us.

Signs Of Chemical Disturbances:

All the functional or physiological processes of life are chemical reactions and are directly related to the chemical inputs received from the mouth, nose, and skin. Though the reactions inside are also affected by mental and genetic makeup, the first and easiest way is to regulate the inputs through food, air, and skin exposure.

Don't neglect the indigestion signals, change in appetite or bowel movements, and discomfort inside the body's parts like chest, head, and abdomen — which are the earliest indicators. If analyzed immediately, we will understand the cause, and simple action can prevent the further progress of it becoming a disease.

For example, if one develops an upset stomach after a heavy meal in a function, it makes sense to have a very light next meal or even skip it rather than resorting to some medicines. Won't it make sense to avoid alcohol, and instead take an antacid and anti-vomiting pills when you feel you have eaten a lot?

Signs Of Disturbances In Energy Processes:

Inability to concentrate on existing work, wanting to take a break often, lack of enthusiasm, fatigue, temporary weakening of hand and finger grip, and inability to stand for long periods, frequently sighing, and irritability signal the disturbances in your energy process. When you notice these symptoms, it is better to take a break and rest for a while, rather than pushing to your limits – it can damage the internal mechanisms leading to neurological diseases. We can improve our energy levels with certain consistent practices. Pranayama, Yoga, and other relaxation techniques go a long way.

Signs Of Disturbances In Mental And Emotional Processes:

The feeling of being lonely, worried, angry, frustrated, helpless, jealous, self-pity, and cruel are all signs of emotional disturbance. Most of these signs show up due to long term practices, and it is tough even to identify them. These are all sudden natural reactions. However, they can be avoided by self-analysis using intellect, rather than analyzing others' faults or situations.

The untrained intellect tries to justify our behavior and rationalize our actions. Avoid this trap by concentrating only on self-correction and improvement always, and with a detached mind. It becomes very simple to avoid these emotional disturbances when practiced.

Emotional disturbances are the root cause of all lifestyle diseases and also lead to relationship issues and conflicts. The way forward is the harmonious balancing of all the processes of life. The foremost important step in this journey is by identifying yourself. The source of health is you.

You are the 'Inergy,' the intelligence-driven energy.

We lead our lives in search of happiness and peace.

Your identity is with this 'Inergy,' not with your body. Your body is only a gadget for usage, and you are way beyond this.

All the problems arise because of our misidentification with the body. Whatever we identify with, we become that.

If you identify with the Inergy, made of happiness and peace, you will not create problems out of incidents, issues, and situations but use them for your benefits.

All your identities with your body and its extensions like name and fame, positions and professions, possessions, and passions. They are not you.

Start your day by reminding, repeating, reciting, and rejoicing with your new identity of 'Inergy,' made of happiness and peace.

The source of health is you, the outcome of Inergy is happiness and peace, and the embodiment of Inergy is health.

Achievement and maintenance of health are not to be confused with checking and chasing ever-expanding physical and chemical parameters. Their role is very peripheral and can only detect disease processes at an earlier stage.

We should concentrate only on our life processes, irrespective of 'normal' parameters. Health is the resultant. This is the way forward from believing, to be happy, to becoming happiness and peace.

Happiness Personified Is The Key To Health.

The physical, chemical, and intelligence processes of life and its role play in our health are discussed in a simplified manner in this book to guide the individuals towards their goal. The fourth dimension of life, the spiritual process is beyond this book's scope and hopefully will be talked about in the next DIY/SIY series.

I reached my clinic and opened the envelope, which said 'Raja.' It was a letter from Resource. There were two papers in the envelope. A love letter was addressing me and a sheet of 'Ten Commandments.' I opened the letter and started reading it.

The Letter Read,

"Hi Source, let me be frank with you. It was not at all a great experience interacting with you. I hope I will not get this sort of opportunity again!" it read; my face turned pale. I could not tell what went wrong!

There was a knock on the door, and before I could see who it was, somebody entered inside. It was a final year medical student. He had come to me as he was unable to pass stools for the past two days. He was in severe pain. I put on my gloves and did a check. I could sense something hard, and it did not feel normal. When I enquired further, he told me that he was trying to clean the inside of his rectum thoroughly using shampoo and that the shampoo bottle had slipped out of his hand and went inside the rectum! He expected me to believe this. I nodded as I did not want to embarrass him further. Later I took him into Operation theatre and, by ingenious means, removed it under local anesthesia. I advised him not to do that sort of perversion activity again.

After reaching home, I hesitantly opened his letter and continued reading it. Hi Source, "Let me be frank with you. It was not at all a great experience interacting with you. I hope I will not get this sort of opportunity again." I read it again. I was disappointed. I felt like throwing the letter away. However, I swallowed my anger and continued reading the letter.

Resource went on to say, "Meeting you was a life-changing event, a divine intervention. I regret not having met you earlier. I can't tell you how invaluable the sessions were. I really can't put a price on the limitless time, knowledge shared, and sincerity you have shown towards me. I want to give this accompanying chart, on which I am sure you will weave your magic to create the book for transforming the lives of millions, especially the millennials." I was surprised and thrilled to read this.

Expectations:

How they influence our minds despite so much knowledge and practice! How much automated are our reactions? But other practice and patience will bring us back to sanity, before taking any precipitative actions!

Whenever we make an observation, wait a minute before making an opinion. After the opinion, confirm your findings, which may be heresy or illusory. Having established the truth, wait for some time before judging people. Then mull all the possible corrective actions to be taken. Then take necessary action without any ill will against any person. Then you are saved from your own anger and fury. If we closely analyze in all our issues, we are primarily responsible, though we feel somebody has cheated or disobeyed us.

You noticed that many papers are piled up on your boss's table, and you arranged them properly.

Your first level of expectation is that he will appreciate you. It didn't happen; you overcame your first level and continued your job.

Your second level of expectation was, at least he is happy because he is not objecting. But later, he showed his annoyance. Still, you continued happily overcoming the third level of expectations. Then your boss attributed motives for arranging the papers to impress him. You were stopped to do it. You stopped doing it, but still, you were not perturbed by his false accusation or biased opinion, as you have overcome your fourth and final level of expectations. Now you are the master!

I was reading the letter, but I couldn't help but wonder where Resource could be at the moment. He had walked away and was not traceable. I was yearning to tell him that I was the one who was inspired and transformed from a 'knowledge imprisoned doctor' to a free-minded wiser human.

With that thought, I opened the 'Ten Commandments,' went through them, absorbed the essence, and started sharing it with those who would need it.

The Ten Commandments:

- Diseases do not discriminate between rich and poor. So, there should not be any bias in the way patients are treated.
- Health is not just wealth. It is everything one can ask for. If you have health, you can face any demon all by yourself.
- You are not your body, but "intelligent internal energy" or 'Inergy,' as I call it, a part of the cosmic energy.
- Life is a synchronized process of physical, chemical, energy, and intelligence.
- You are responsible for your health. Everything else is secondary.
- The Source of all diseases is in mind, so is the cure.
- Lifestyle diseases are the result of our ignorance. However, it can be reversed with proper knowledge and practice.
- The choice of treatment options – the kind of treatment, whom to consult, which hospital to trust, and all this is decided by intuition, not merely by gathered information. Choose wisely!
- The surgical, medicinal, and mental health approach to treat the diseases is needed, but incomplete, inadequate, and temporary.
- Health is not a mere absence of diseases or maintenance of parameters. It also has its dynamics.

Rapid-fire:

I imagined what questions I would have asked and how he would have replied.

1. What is life?
"Nothing but thoughts released from the collected data."
2. How is data of thoughts created?
"From our actions and intentions."
3. How to make life happy, peaceful, and healthy?
"By creating happy, peaceful, and useful thoughts."
4. What are the parameters of health?
"Being happy, enthusiastic, active, lively, trusting, and harmonious."

EPILOGUE

Last week — Twenty years later, I was trying to reduce my patient load by delegating them to junior doctors and posting a receptionist at the entrance to filter unwanted guests.

Resource somehow gatecrashed and dropped into my chamber of the new, bigger hospital, without the help of a borrowed stethoscope around his neck. Probably bribed the receptionist with American chocolates.

This time we instantly recognized each other, despite greying and losing hair on the head, growing of beard and mustache, because we were both in our childhood level of consciousness. Nothing to lose, nothing to gain. Avoided 'shake hands' and greeted each other by Indian way, 'Namaste.'

He explained his sudden unannounced disappearance from the scene. Except for a slight Indo-American accent, his attitude remained the same.

He had met a companion online, flew off to California, refused reinstatement in his software company as vice president, and after a variety of 'resourceful' odd jobs, in the country of opportunity, started writing books on topics which he little understood and became a celebrity and found out the formula and art of book writing, started his own publishing company. He was tracking me, from wherever he was, as I was a sitting duck. He came to fulfill his prophecy, to make me write a book or two or even ten.

He started telling me about me why and how to write a book. I surprised him by showing the prototype I had written.

DR. RAJASEKHAR RAMAKRISHNA MYSORE

He offered to edit and publish it for me.

We met the next day at the same restaurant, a cafe, with a grand ambiance and prices. As we waited for our coffee to arrive, Resource started narrating his story:

"Dude, I met Shirin, a US citizen of Iranian origin." A broad smile came on to my face. He didn't understand why. He continued, "I met her on Facebook. For the first time in my forty years of existence, stunning looks, I was attracted by the opposite sex. It is still a mystery why she accepted my 'friend request.' Instantly we liked each other on Facebook. I flew to California, where she was residing. No doubt, I recognized her with difficulty as the face I had seen on Facebook was when she was twenty years old. But at 42 still, she was beautiful though not stunning. In one way, I was happy that she was okay with me, despite my looks."

Accepting the age-old idiom 'Marriages are made in Heaven,' we solemnized our marriage in a combination of Hindu and Persian wedding styles.

'Deja Vu,' a smile popped up again, he won't understand, I thought.

"It was too late to bear children, so we enjoyed a prolonged honeymoon. She is a journalist. I worked as an assistant for her for some time until I decided what to do. I attended Shiv Khera's seminars (smile on my face again), worked in Raam Anand's publishing company, and now on my own. Do you know why I came to India? Just to meet you. I want my first real book to be authored by you. Till now, I was into children's books, comics, educational tips, etc."

"How about your personal life? Why were you smiling big when I was narrating mine? Was that funny?"

I laughed again and started, "When I start my post-graduation story, you will know why I was smiling."

I finished my Master's in general surgery from Kurnool Medical college in 1984, married Chandrika in May. She was doing her post-graduation in Gynecology. Three months later, I went to Iran and my friends Achuth and Sarathi, for a job in the ministry of health. There was a lot of advice against going to Iran as there was a war between Iran and Iraq.

You know, I am the person who won't go back, having taken a decision. It was a friendly country. Persian culture was great, unlike what we had thought of before. They are hardworking, intelligent, smart, and very courteous people. They love India, Hindi films, and our celebrations. But they were unable to understand that human beings can survive on a vegetarian diet. 😊

Now you know why I smiled when you told me about your wife. I continued as he showed interest. My first posting was in Ilam, about 30 km from the border with Iraq. I was advised to request a transfer as it was one of the most dangerous areas. I refused and joined.

Daily anti-aircraft guns booming and sirens warning imminent attacks were a regular event. After a month, I got transferred to a safer place due to local politics. Two months later, my wife joined me, notwithstanding the war. I consider that as a courageous decision. She stayed in Tehran alone for a week to take an exam before getting a job.

Tehran was fortified with anti-aircraft and anti-missile guns and a lot of sandbags surrounding the buildings. Iraq had superior air power and Iran dedicated manpower. The war lasted the entire period of our stay for almost ten years. Coffins of martyrs being taken in a procession were regular in every city.

Now you know why I smiled when you mentioned your Iranian connection. We had funny encounters with the Persian language, which was alien to us. The other smile was when you mentioned Shiv Khera, 'You Can Win' is the book I recommended to all youngsters and continue to do so even now. Why don't you come home and join us for lunch tomorrow?

"See, Sekhar, I learned the concept of our identities, detachment, relationships, etc., from you. Let our friendship be on this plane only." "He has gone a step ahead of me," I thought. He made his trademark comment:

"Wow! The most evolved, most intelligent species is being

threatened out of its existence by the least evolved, tiniest living organism on earth."

"THE CORONA!"

"How's that?"

I just smiled.

"Then...what are your discoveries of life?" Resource questioned. He was partly teasing and partly serious.

I declared, "Live to your fullest potential."

"To enjoy health, we must experience life differently."

I will discuss the following subjects more elaborately to start practicing the conclusions we have come to.

"Go ahead. I will record on my mobile app," he started.

FOOD

Let's begin with the most fundamental aspect of our lives: food and nutrition. Food is one of the essential ingredients for survival, sustenance, and growth. So, it is considered divine.

Food is eaten when hungry, for taste, for fun, even when angry, for 'time pass,' or because it is available free.

DIET

If one selects food items with a particular quantity, at a particular time or particular variety, for a specific purpose, it is called diet — for example, vegetarian vs. nonvegetarian; high calorie vs. low calorie; one meal vs. multiple meals.

NUTRITION is the science of the food, for health and growth. It is the science of ingredients in food for health and growth. There are four gross components and some micro components in the food we eat.

1. Carbohydrates: These are present in single grain products (monocotyledons) like rice, wheat, maize, oats, ragi, millets, etc. After digestion, all these will be converted into glucose in the intestines. Glucose is the energy giver for all the cells in the body. Every activity in the cells, tissues, organs, and systems in the body requires a continuous supply of glucose. All physical and mental activities by the body also require glucose.

Which is the best source? Rice or wheat or millers or oats? None of them is superior or inferior. Whole grains, least processed, locally available, or grown and used from childhood, are ideal for individuals. Excess of carbohydrates consumed and not used for physical activities will be converted to fat and preserved, and when glucose is not available, it will be converted back from fat. But this is a tedious process, and some undesirable by-products will be produced.

2. Proteins: Are the building blocks of all cells. So for growth and replacement of dead tissue, proteins are needed. They are derived from animal meat or poultry or dicotyledons like beans, lentils, grams, etc. All the proteins will be broken down into amino acids for absorption in the intestines. Protein needs are slightly more during pregnancy, in growing children, and in vigorous exercises for bodybuilding. Again, excess protein intake, when not needed, will be converted to fat. If sufficient glucose is not available, protein breaks down for glucogenesis. Again, the by-products are harmful.

3. Fat and oils: At room temperature, if the fat is in liquid form, it is called oil. About 15 to 20 grams of oil is required for the absorption of specific fat-soluble vitamins. The rest of the fat will give double the energy compared to carbs or proteins. Excess fat gets accumulated in different organs like the liver, pancreas, kidneys, and blood vessels are harmful to the body.

4. Fibre or roughage: Fibre, both soluble and insoluble, are required for the formation of stools. Nonvegetarian sources of food do not have enough fiber. They also have a role in the absorption of certain elements of food.

5. Micronutrients: vitamins, minerals, gut microbiota. A minimal quantity of vitamins and minerals in micrograms is needed for the maintenance of the body. Now the significance of bacteria in the gut is being explored, and its role in maintaining normal health is appreciated.

1. All this general knowledge about food is only for information.
2. How to use this knowledge for regular food intake is more important. You just can't measure everything in each meal and consume scientifically.

There Are Two Ways Of Eating Food For Health.

1. Those who follow a disciplined, ritualistic lifestyle must eat varieties of food, including almost equal quantities of carbs, vegetable proteins (lentils, dals, beans), and vegetables: a spoon or two of fat or oil. The measurement is not by weight but by visual measures like a cup or bowl. A cup of curds/yogurt and a glass of milk. A sour fruit like orange, lemon, mango, amla, etc. in a small quantity in the uncooked form, For example, whole fruit or in pickle form, which gives vitamin C (which gets destroyed at 60 degrees centigrade of temperature). Different varieties of vegetables, including greens, are to be rotated each day.
2. People who eat nonvegetarian food predominantly must eat plenty of vegetable salads and liquid food like soups.
3. An occasional sweet or fried item or pastries or chocolate or ice cream (taste-based food) can be added once a week for fun. Indulgence in this sort of food is to be strictly avoided.
4. Regarding the quantity of food, the lesser, the better. If your stomach feels full after a meal, it indicates overeating. Be aware of that and cut down on the next meal. If you feel lethargic sometimes after a meal, it shows gluttony, not a digestive issue!
5. In general, all those who are in normal to just above average weight range are eating at least double the

quantity than required, and somehow the system struggles to clear that excess, and that's the reason for the postprandial lethargy.

Those who don't go by the clock for their food should follow the signals from their system like hunger, craving certain food types. Such folks don't give much importance to varieties or taste. They just follow the body's needs.

The third type of people who indulge in eating, also known as foodies, who eat for every occasion and no reason have overruled their sensors and senses for long. They need strong motivation, determination, and medical and psychological help.

Obesity is not a simple abnormality. Morbid obesity is a dangerous disease and requires urgent medical intervention.

Psychological Management Of Eating Habits:

1. The way we eat food is also important. Don't simply gulp the food. Eat in a calm, pleasant atmosphere. When food is eaten in a hurry, and stress will carry those emotions into our minds. Digestion will also be affected.

2. Food, while eating, should be considered a gift from nature, and our ability to digest and assimilate is a blessing. We must also remember that we are among the minuscule population, and the majority in the world, including children, don't get two meals a day.

3. Overeating is also a type of wasting of this divine commodity. If we are obese, it means we have eaten somebody' else's food. While eating, be aware of how much and what you are eating; and beware of indulgence.

Enjoy every morsel of food irrespective of its taste. Each person's taste is a developed habit and not by nature, as many believe. It can be changed by practice. There are thousands of different flavors and try to accept each as something unique.

Don't describe the food as 'I love it' or 'I hate it.' I like it, or I don't like it. Day to day food need not be an elaborate course of the meal. Variation in tastes, flavors are normal. Don't try to standardize food items like, "Dosa should be crispier," etc. After eating food, don't discuss how nice it was. We have to get it again, where is it available, that particular place is great for taste, etc. Just forget about it. These are the types of thoughts that make food as a pleasure and not as a necessity. Don't watch food shows on TV or online. The addiction to food starts from there. It is as dangerous as drug addiction, if not more.

Those who want to reduce weight must consider food as a necessary evil. Unfortunately, obesity is not out of ignorance. Most of them know diet, nutritional values, etc. They must start telling themselves that they hate sweets and high-calorie food. Though, in the beginning, it looks that we are fooling ourselves, it is better than being fooled by our minds, the accumulated past thoughts. In three to four weeks, you will see the results.

Water:

How much? When? Whenever you feel thirsty. When your lips and tongue are dry, urine becomes dark in color and less in quantity (a sign of dehydration). If you feel too thirsty, drinking too much water and passing urine in large quantities and frequently suspect and exclude diabetes. Too much of anything is bad, including water.

Digestion and absorption of food depend on the mood with which you are eating. Eat calmly, happily, and without any distractions like the TV, Mobile, Laptop, music, discussions, arguments, and debates. Dedicate those few minutes for eating only.

Eating is an art, not science. How many times to chew, when to drink water before, during, or after food are secondary. There's one more concept about the intake of food. The food we eat not only carries the chemical ingredients but also some sort of energy called vibrations, that is, the food we eat not only carries the chemical ingredients but along with it some sort of energy called vibrations which will affect our thought processes. So starting from preparation to preserving to consuming, there are certain processes to be followed, which will give us overall benefits. Like the concept of a sattvic diet, wherein food that is very spicy and irritable is avoided. Food of only vegetarian origin and only milk from cows is allowed. While preparing food, it should be done with a pious mind and serene background so that the food carries similar emotions into our mind. It may not be able to prove this, but by observation, we can appreciate it.

To Summarise,
    a. Lesser the better;
    b. More varieties the better,
    c. Eat enthusiastically, not excitedly.

Sleep

With food covered, let's get to sleep. We know that humans experience three phases of sleep, wakeful state, dream state, and deep sleep state. In a wakeful state, the body, mind, and intellect are active. During a dream state, the only mind is working, physical and intellectual components are subdued. In the deep sleep state, all the major components are subdued, but the innate intelligence is active, and all subconscious activities are functioning efficiently.

So, sleep is not a state where a gadget is simply turned off. In the wakeful state, though the physical activity is very obvious, it is still the projection of our mental activity through thoughts.

In the dream state, the physical and intellectual components are subdued, but we still feel that the dream is real. We feel the same fear, excitement, anxiety, etc. as in the wakeful state. We can't even make out that it is a dream. But when it is too scary, we wake up with the help of innate intelligence.

If we closely analyze this concept, we learn that during the dream state, we see everything with eyes closed and are hearing without the help of ears. So, even during the wakeful state, it is the mind's interpretation of the data, received from eyes, ears, nose, skin and tongue and other sensations from many other parts of the body that we are experiencing as real.

During the deep sleep state, we are completely oblivious to our life. So, it is this state of deep sleep that is real, wherein we are most peaceful, pleasant, and happy, without any interference from our mind. That is the state we crave for, but our mind forces us to wake up and pushes us into the wakeful state, to perpetuate our daily activities. When it gets exhausted, slowly, it reverts home to the deep sleep state. During the deep sleep state, three things happen.

Firstly, we go to our original state for some time, experiencing real happiness and peace. The internal energy recharges itself, and the innate intelligence works hard to relieve us of pains and help us rest. In a nutshell, the wakeful state of around 16 hours a day is the superimposition of our mind using sensory organs of the body. Think of sleep as a home screen of all our activities. It is our original state. When the physical and mental processes subside, then sleep starts its job of recharging the energy. Sleep is neither a sin nor a waste of our precious time. It enhances our experiences and the efficiency of our wakeful activities. Deficient or excess sleep are both harmful to healthy living

Furthermore, we always wonder how to get sleep? Here's the thing, you can't get sleep. It is already there. You simply have to allow the physical and mental activities to recede. Whenever you decide to sleep, retract all your senses: close your eyes, ignore all sounds, smell, etc. Switch off the lights.

But the most important thing is to switch off the mind. It takes more time to turn off the mind than to close the eyes or switch off the lights. So, before going to bed, do not stimulate your mind with emotions, especially from audio-visual media. Avoid watching the news, texting, or having a conversation on the phone. Calming music with repetitive tunes may help in closing the apps in the mind. However, it's advisable that you actively try and sleep.

Older people may require less sleep during the night because their energy recharging needs are not high. It would help them if they simply lay down and thought good things. A heavy, late meal may cause physical discomfort or delay in falling asleep. Avoid tiring yourself to the point of exhaustion and then falling asleep because this is like a computer crashing because it is overheated.

Similarly, taking medicines or drinking to fall asleep is like forcing the system to shut down. These substances have a negative effect on the body. We can see that going to sleep is like shutting down a computer. Close all tabs one by one, allow the system to check and close. A little time is required for the process.

A person needs a minimum of four hours of intense deep-sleep every day to function well. You'll know you are well-rested when you wake up fresh the next morning and do not have body aches, irritability, or drowsiness. Your day will go better. You won't be complaining and lethargic.

To maintain your health, try not to oversleep as well. You'll know you have overslept if your day starts slowly, and you are lethargic.

Exercise

With food and sleep covered, let's get to exercise. It is primarily of two types: routine and scheduled. We know that all creatures in the wild do not schedule their exercise, and yet they are fit. Likewise, humans were considered to be physically active about 40 years ago by just doing routine activities. Using public transport and fetching water from the well-made humans healthy and fit. In fact, all the previous generations needed was a bit of evening walking, and they were good to go, unlike today, where youngsters are advised to get off their desks and stretch every 30 minutes because their backs and lower limbs seem to be wasting away.

Thanks to technology, everything is easily available, and this has made the younger generation lazy. Now, they need gyms, personal trainers and whatnot to stay fit. Our body can be understood as the hardware of a gadget, which needs regular maintenance. If any part of the body is not used regularly, then it becomes weak and finally non-functional. So, we have no choice but to be physically active just to keep this machine running.

Whether to do it as a matter of routine like taking stairs instead of the lift, walking to a grocery shop rather than ordering online, and cooking instead of ordering on mobile apps; or pay and do exercises at fitness centers is your choice.

You can also do Yoga Asanas to help you with posture and peace of mind. Yoga also ensures the physical, physiological, and mental balance. Bending the body into different postures makes all the joints flexible, stretches stiff ligaments, and makes muscles supple. In each posture, the body is bent and maintained in that pose for a certain period. This will stop or reduce blood flow to a particular organ for a short while. And what follows is a relaxation state, where the blood flows back to the organ. The asanas are designed to cover all the organs in the body. Once learned, they can be practiced anywhere without the need for any gadgets. It hardly requires 15 to 20 minutes a day. And unlike exercises, they don't cause exhaustion and don't need nutritional supplements. They make us more active and energetic.

The third effect is mental or spiritual. The word yoga means connection. The connection is between physical and metaphysical. There are many types of Yoga to connect known to the unknown, using body, mind, intellect, or inner energy. Yoga with some sort of exercise is required for all of us today to keep our body and mind balanced.

The type of exercise can be decided by the individual depending on their interest. One may opt for sports or swimming or a brisk walk or running or dance, etc. Yoga or exercises, when done under the sun, will help you get vitamin D and connect you with nature. In order to rejuvenate your respiratory system, you can always do breathing exercises called the Pranayama.

My colleague's husband, who is in his 30s, developed severe hypertension and diabetes despite his wife knowing yoga. Mental stress, coupled with lethargy, makes it hard for you to workout. It is important to know that having the knowledge alone won't yield; only practice makes it possible.

Then there is meditation; it's a deeper process of acquiring knowledge about fundamental doubts or dilemmas directly from the cosmic source without depending on humans. It is essentially a deeper dissection of the concept to be explored by the concentration of intellect on that particular subject, without the involvement of individuals like me, she, he, you.

The process should be non-judgmental, and the ultimate answer should be universally applicable for all times. Meditation is an experience in itself that needs to be experienced by the person.

Lifestyle

"What is a lifestyle? It is such a loosely used word without knowing the real impact of it." Resource confessed. Good, let us discuss this way.

Life processes, though grossly remain the same, each one makes use of it differently. Over a period of time, one gets used to that sort of living, which we can call as his lifestyle.

I have observed that basically, there are three types of lifestyles, one of them one adapts and later modifies depending on his experiences.

They are
1. Disciplined and ritualistic
2. Free and individualistic
3. Vagabond.

None of these are superior or inferior. Each one has its own pros and cons.

Disciplined lifestyle

Usually, this method is learned or imposed from childhood by parents or teachers. The motivation comes from the appreciation one receives and the benefits one sees from their idols or role models one creates in their minds.

It will be considered as an ideal way of living. This lifestyle, once adapted and perfected, makes their day to day lives easy and smooth.

This type of living is dictated mainly by
1. Time
2. The prescribed format in which actions are performed
3. Pride in following that path.

Time

Punctuality is the keyword here. There is a time for any activity to be performed. The clock is the master. Starting from wake-up time to going to bed and almost all activities in between, are time driven. This is, or this is not the time to do, this work is the dictum. They idolize a person, father, mother, a leader, a teacher, etc. and try to follow their way.

Format

Everything has a place; every activity has a method; everybody has a particular role in each activity and responsible for their roles.

The life pattern will be more or less ritualistic and idealistic. The formats are amendable but strictly to be adhered to. There will be formats for everything under the sun, the way to sit, eat, study, talk, drink, sleep. The relationship is of master/slave. The master being the format and the slaves are individuals.

Advantages of this lifestyle

Predictable outcomes, organized flow of work, streamlined activities, and easy for administration.

Predictable outcomes: father brings milk from the booth on his way back for home after his morning walk, which he will not miss a single day. Breakfast will be ready by 8:00 AM; the mother takes care of it. Son wears his shoes by 8:25 AM and starts his vehicle at 8:28 AM to go to his office.

The organized flow of work: Father gets up 5:00 AM, finishes his bath by 5:30 AM, the son takes a bath by 5:40, followed by mother at 5:50 AM. By that time, the father has prepared hot coffee for all.

Streamlined activities: Father reads the Newspaper at 6:00 AM, before leaving for a morning walk. The mother goes through it at noon. Son scans it at night.

The ease of administration is obvious. It works well in organizations with hierarchy and designated responsibilities. Those who are brought up in this lifestyle will be able to work very well in organizations with fixed timings like 9:00 to 5:00 jobs and defined responsibilities.

They are likely to develop hypertension, anxiety, and cardiac problems as their lifestyle diseases, as they can't adjust to changes in the work pattern. For example, many managers in public sector organizations developed health issues when work ethics changed drastically due to globalization.

Disadvantages: Individually, it works wonders if they simply follow it as a way of life, but brings pressure on others who do not adhere to that philosophy. It creates expectations from others and can lead to conflicts. Individual freedom of thoughts will be suppressed. It encourages the status quo, and innovations will be discouraged.

Free lifestyle

Here the individuals have an open mind, explore possibilities, and give preference to results rather than processes. The time frame will be flexible though the overall timeline will be managed. Smarter solutions will emerge. Individual freedom will be there within a framework. Responsibility will be happily shared. A team spirit is required.

Disadvantages:

Results may be unpredictable. Targets may not be met. Those who follow this lifestyle are likely to develop obesity, addictions, and relationship issues, as they are used to follow their mind, not others' expectations.

Vagabond lifestyle:

They have no agenda, no path, no direction in life. They just live from day-to-day. They don't give much importance to files, regulations, morals, ethics, and others' opinions. They don't even have their own ideas. They just live on others' money. They are likely to develop criminal attitudes or commit suicide. Few of them may turn to spirituality.

"Then, which is the best lifestyle?" Resource enquired.

During childhood, when children have not yet developed their own individuality if they are trained in a disciplined lifestyle with parents doing most of it, it is ideal. Later, as they grow, gradual flexibility is allowed to develop their own personality. As they become adults guiding them as and when required, without any expectations from them, will be ideal. A sort of carrot and stick policy may be required in childhood so that they will not suffer in their future.

"A disciplined personal lifestyle for the body, relatively free lifestyle for the mind, and a vagabond lifestyle in spirituality." Resource exclaimed!

Thoughts

The previous night I was contemplating about why, how, and where we get the thoughts? How to streamline them?

The mind releases thoughts for action. After being filtered by the intellect, one of the thoughts is converted into action.

Whenever we act, it produces two effects. One is the physical effect of the action.

For example, you have written a letter to your boss.

"Sir, I always feel you are my inspiration to me. Your work ethics are to be emulated by many. Despite your high position, you are a very humble person and very humane. You are known in the whole organization for helping employees whenever needed. As you know, I am having personal problems at home, and I am aware it is a 'project launch time' in the office. I request you to grant me one month's leave from next Monday."

This is the physical part of your action. But you know that your boss is just the opposite of what you have mentioned in the letter. The intention part of your action was to somehow get the leave sanctioned.

The intentions are recorded in the data bank, the mind. Similar intentions repeated over many times will start releasing as thoughts of duplicity. You start doing the same thing with your friends, family. You start thinking that you are very smart.

Though it looks that thoughts released by the mind are spontaneous, they are actually from the data bank we have created by our actions.

So, for everyone, the different thoughts released spontaneously from their minds are from the data banks they have created by their repeated actions.

If you always want happy thoughts in your mind, you can't try to manage at the thought level. You have to do it at an action level.

Do every action you are doing in any given role happily.

They will be recorded as happy thoughts and released as happy thoughts for any future actions you are assigned.

For instance, your junior has not come to work. You have to do his job, which you feel as inferior. So you are doing it unhappily, and it gets recorded as unhappiness in your data bank and later released as unhappy thoughts. You start feeling unhappiness, for no reason. Similarly, your assistant doesn't want or can't meet your expectations; you are frustrated. Those frustrations get into your data bank, and your frustrations start showing on everybody, everywhere.

Resource was not convinced and countered, "But how can we imagine happiness or peace when the facts are opposite?"

"Yes, initially, it looks very artificial. But if you carefully observe, you will notice two issues here. One is your expectations from yourself or others. Expectations are yours, and only you can reduce them and overcome them. Later you can plan for correcting or improving others. The second issue is identification and attachment to the roles you play. Your identity is with your inner energy, 'the Inergy.' You being 'the boss' is only a temporary role, don't get attached to it. You are not the boss, you play the role of the boss in your office, and you can also play the role of an assistant when required." I replied.

Become a good actor by playing the given role well and come out of it.

A great actor never identifies with any particular role; he just plays the role to his best and comes out of it. For example, Amitabh Bachchan is given a guest role, even just for a minute, where he delivers a single dialogue in such a way that we remember that dialogue forever, even though we forget the movie itself.

So, playing the role well to the best of our ability, irrespective of the given role is more important than the role itself.

Roles simply come on our way, though we feel we have chosen them. All the positions we get or hold in our lives, be it in personal, professional, or social lives, are all simply temporary roles. We are neither those positions nor those of our identities.

Our role in getting roles is very minimal. Just understand that everyone is playing the role assigned to them in this big opera.

So, to reverse diabetes, for example, the process is simple.

There are five principles to get rid of diabetes: diet, exercise, medicines, investigations, and mind management.

If the sugars are above the normal limits, start all the processes of diabetic management. Start following medicines prescribed by your doctor, do exercises to reduce weight and increase the utilization of sugars, follow the diet as advised by your doctor or dietician, get regular check-ups of your physical and blood parameters as advised according to your blood sugar levels.

The last and the most important one is mind management for a stress-free life, which you should continue for life. It will be your way of life for happiness and peace. As the reversal starts, your medicines will be reduced gradually and stopped ultimately, if you practice all the other processes regularly and happily.

If the blood sugars are just above normal limits, hoping to wish it away by half-hearted attempts and ill-conceived methods will not help. Except for medicines, all four other principles of diabetes management should be started earnestly and at the earliest under the guidance of your doctor. Mind management is the most important principle which is being discussed now.

The Flow Chart For Your Mind Management Is Like This.

1. Your identity is with the INERGY, the inner intelligence-driven energy, also known as you.
2. Your identity with the body is to be deleted, and your relationship with the body is to be considered as that of ownership. The body is yours, but not YOU.
3. All the diseases are caused by our different emotional excesses like avarice, greed, arrogance, jealousy, etc.
4. Emotions are nothing but thoughts contaminated by 'I, me, mine,' the self-centered feelings vs. the others.
5. Thoughts are released from memory in mind, which are formed from our repeated actions with emotions.
6. So, if we perform all our actions happily, peacefully, usefully, purposefully, with a sense of detachment, they

will be recorded as happy, peaceful, useful, purposeful, and divine thoughts. Similar thoughts will be released for actions. This cycle of great thoughts and actions perpetuate.
7. Life is nothing but our thoughts. With all positive, happy, and peaceful thoughts pouring in, life becomes happy and peaceful.

This Happiness Is The Source And Manifestation Of Health.

Relationships /friendships

Relationships At Different Levels:

First, the relationship between 'I,' the 'Inergy,' and my body, as a master and slave, should be well established. Then, all the other relationships are with my body and mind, with other bodies and minds. Relationships with my parents, wife, children, and siblings are through my body. Other relationships and friendships are through my mind with their minds.

"Though we give a lot of hype to those friendships emotionally, it's as good as pressing the accept or reject button of a friendship request on Facebook." Resource said.

Friendships are developed with emotional connectivity to others with some commonality, like classmates, the same professionals, common interests, etc. But a really intense and intimate, or lasting friendship is when the thought processes of the individuals are in sync with one another. But all these are emotional attachments and should be understood from that perspective. All emotional attachments are associated with the pain-pleasure cycles.

Habits:

Why do we develop habits, and how to change when required? Habit is an automated release of thoughts, resulting in actions. These will help us in saving time and energy for performing repetitive or cyclic functions.

Useful habits are called good habits, and harmful habits are bad habits. Habits when they defy logic it is compulsive behavior. Habits that give pleasure but are harmful and difficult to reverse are an addiction.

For elaboration, we take an example of watching a program on your mobile. Morning once you get up, you start a devotional song on your app for 15 minutes, followed by your routine. It gives you a pleasant day. It becomes a habit. Due to any reason, if that could not happen for a few days, you will feel something lacking. Then you forget about it after three weeks.

Then you start going for a game, and you get some appreciation. After some time, you get habituated to it as it gives some physical benefits and appreciation. So, to stop it becomes more difficult unless you replace it with similar activity. You start seeing a porn video. It gives you excitement. You continue doing it. You get addicted to it.

You start consuming alcohol as a socializing factor. But gradually you get habituated to it. But still, you may have control over it. But if you face an unforeseen catastrophe in life, this same habit can become addictive as it gives an escape route from facing reality.

Habits can be developed as a useful tool, like physical exercises every day, meditation; for time management (waking up and going to bed at a designated time). But for any habit, we should not become a slave. So, all those good habits are also to be given a break once in a while, so that we do not become dependent on it. We must be aware of our habits and have control over it.

My friend, Narayan, who is a runner and participates in many marathons on a regular basis, was advised to reduce it, as his heart rate was going down to dangerously low levels during his sleep.

The analogy is like using your mobile phone. You set to-wake-up alarms, reminders in the calendar — these are useful apps or habits. Every day at a particular time, you are using a music app. After some time, you start getting reminders for that app. Later it will add some ads to lure you. Then you must be alert; otherwise, you are likely to land in problems.

Similarly, with smoking, alcohol, drugs, it starts as a style or status symbol due to peer pressure. It is also defended as 'just for the company' or 'social drinking.' The basic process starts as a thought, introduced from outside, like media, pressure groups, icons, cinemas, social parties, etc. It will be recorded as a norm or even great.

Thoughts work by the release of chemicals in the brain. Repeated release of chemicals will form neuronal pathways, which will form reflexes, thereby causing circuits.at this level, it becomes difficult to reverse habits as they are already automated. At later stages, there will be permanent physical changes in the brain. Then it is called addiction, and it will be extremely difficult to reverse it.

Some chemicals are called neuro stimulants; they directly affect the brain bypassing the thought process. They are called 'drugs,' and people who are addicted to them are 'drug addicts.' They not only cause addictive changes in the brain but also cause changes that blunt intellect, memory, emotions, morality. This is a disease, not a psychological variation or aberration. Their brain needs a continuous supply of those substances for their mental survival. And many times, it will be irreversible

The patient, family, and society have to pay the price for it. So, Substance abuse should be curtailed by whatever means. But the best way is to prevent it by awareness programs and educating at homes and schools and especially colleges and by demonizing it.

There is one more new addiction, which is equally dangerous. That is Internet Addiction; it includes gaming apps, pornography, extremist ideologies, irresponsible freedom. They are causing havoc in the lives of highly intelligent youth and destroying their careers.

Rapes, child abuse, domestic violence, workplace abuse, exploitation, etc. are some of the offshoots of the thought process anomalies. All these need to be addressed for a healthy society, which everyone is a part of.

A small comment on exhaustion and relaxation, there are two aspects to it. Physical exhaustion is that the body is not able to cope up with the activities performed. If those activities are essential for survival, improve your abilities by a gradual build-up of your muscular strength, or reduce the work. If the exhaustion is mental, the chemicals in the brain need to be replenished by giving small breaks to recover. We are not born to work. We are here to experience life. If you think job or professional work is a necessary evil and so finish it and then go for relaxation or enjoyment, you will have neither of them to its fullest.

JOB, WORK, PROFESSION, GOING OUT, CLUB, TOURS, RESORTS, ENTERTAINMENT, DANCE, SOCIALISING ARE ALL SIMPLY PHYSICAL ACTIVITIES.

The emotional feelings of bugging, tedious, frustrating, fun, enjoyment are all simply thoughts released by the mind. When they are extrapolated, the problems arise, and solutions are evasive.

Knowledge

One of the most misunderstood words is knowledge.

INFORMATION, KNOWLEDGE, WISDOM ARE OFTEN LOOSELY INTERCHANGED.

They are different levels of the same process. Information: inform is only grasping the form. A child learns the alphabet A, B, C... without understanding the significance of it.

That is INFORMATION for the child at that stage. But the child thinks that it 'knows' the alphabet. But when it starts using alphabets in forming sentences, it understands the significance of alphabets. At this stage, the child is in the stage of UNDERSTANDING.

Later it uses sentences for reading and writing, and at this stage, it has KNOWLEDGE. This stage yields limited benefits to the person. After that, the person starts using that knowledge in his day to day transactions, which is WISDOM. At this stage, he gets full benefits.

Most of the younger generation think that information is power. Information itself is not only not useful, but sometimes can be harmful.

Many argue that it is better to collect a lot of information. Those who have a well-trained intellect as a filter can manage excess information. Others will struggle with information because the mind, with all its emotions, plays with the information. Those with balanced minds refuse to collect unnecessary information.

You read on WhatsApp that an Indian was attacked in a city suburb in the USA. Your mind immediately starts working on that piece of information, and your emotions flare up- poor Indian, these American rogues, the complicity of the police, the public are jealous of Indians, I doubt whether NRIs will come to his help, it goes on like that, then is a lot of discussions among your WhatsApp groups producing mass hysteria.

Relatives and friends of all Indians in America start calling them or sending messages, the incident of which they are unaware of.

After a long time, you will come to know that it was 'a native Indian,' not an 'Indian Indian' who was involved. But you already had a fight with your close friend for his different view on that information, because he considered Indians there are arrogant and deserve that sort of treatment.

The simple medical information on the net, about all the modes of spread, brings thousands of people who visited night clubs for HIV testing labs.

"Information is just ingredients, knowledge is half baked information, and wisdom is fully prepared and served food. Relish the wisdom. Curtail unnecessary information," Resource comprehended.

How to decide which information is needed and which is

not?

Ask a simple question, "What role should I play with that information?" If the answer is nothing, just delete it. Don't even forward it. It affects many more people to deal with their already overloaded data.

"The burden of excess information is the looming crisis for health," he quipped and packed up by saying, "bye."

The next session was on DESIRES.

Lord Buddha had concluded 'desires are the root cause of all miseries.' What is your take on that?

In a way, he was correct. It is like the concept of 'birth is the cause of death.' Those are the concepts at a metaphysical level of living. But practically, human existence and progress are only dependent on desires, individual and collective.

Desires to ambitions, to avarice, and catastrophe is the normal path, if not tread properly. Desire is thought for progressing from where we are.

The intention is the next step to achieve the desired. Then comes planning and action. Desires can be general like, 'Let the whole world be happy.' It is also called a wish.

Ambition is the higher level of desire with a strong attachment to 'Me.' It is usually associated with positions like, I want to become a great actor, or I want to become a professor.

Being greedy is the possessiveness of materialistic things with unending satiety. This is the phase where an aura is created around the person. Megalomania develops, leading to a downfall.

An entrepreneur who establishes many successful companies looks invincible with all political coterie. But suddenly, he becomes bankrupt and flees the country. A classic example of greed killing the goose.

How to assess the journey from a desire to ambition to greed? Everyone will have many desires, and most of them will not be converted to intentions.

So, the desires die at that. Many of the intentions die as there is no plan. Most of the plans are shelved as there is no action.

Most of the actions do not fructify due to a lack of commitment. At the level of ambition, answers to a single question will solve the problem.

What Is The Purpose Of Your Ambition?

If the answer is a personal accomplishment, think twice before embarking on it. One of my classmates competed in a competitive exam, got selected for a medical course, completed it, and later, he chose to become a civil contractor. His ambition was to be called a doctor! What a waste of time and a professional seat!

If the purpose of our ambition serves society in a larger context, it is better. If your ambition is to become a leader so that you can wield power, or a spiritual guru to exploit the gullible, your ambition will lead you to disaster. Desires are human, harmless per se, ambitions with only personal agenda are dangerous. Greed is disastrous.

Age

I define age as a change measured in time. Everything that exists changes over a period of time. From the stage of our conception, we are changing.

Applied to life, this process called aging, is in all its different processes. Physically, it is slowly growing and gradually deteriorating.

Functionally, it is gradually improving and gradually slowing. Mentally, it is more undulatory and gradually flattening.

Spiritually it is ever-evolving. So, it is only in the spiritual process that the change is always progressive, even though most of us are unaware of it.

The rate of progress may be different for each one of us.

But all of us are at different levels of spiritual evolution.

Some of us have understood the mechanism and driving at our own pace; the rest of them are being pushed.

If the spiritual process is in our control, the body, its functions, mental processes will have smooth and slow aging.

The key is not in dyeing our hair, botoxing our wrinkles, or wearing clothes like youth. It is not even living in the past by connecting to school mates and imagining youth. It is to become child-like, not childish.

With the least amount of attachments, opinions, and differentiation, acceptance and equanimity are the keys to graceful aging.

The indication of aging is when we start living in the past. Like saying how nice it was in college, those days were different, etc.

Aging starts from the time we stop seeing the future and start living in the past. It is not chronological age that counts, not even biological age but our spiritual age that matters.

"Don't think, count, or bother about your age. Just go ahead," was Resource's summary.

Values In Life

An interesting topic. Values in life are an individual's emotional thoughts developed during the formative years with moral, ethical, religious convictions in the background. They are better when not judged by others; they are more for our own upliftment.

Dilemmas And Confusions

Conflicts in the mind, a crucial topic for day to day life.

A beggar is begging in front of a temple. You have donated x amount to the temple, and you are against giving alms to the poor. Is it right or wrong?

You have invested a large amount in your hospital. A poor patient comes for your treatment. What will you do?

Your personal driver is admitted to the hospital. You ask for a concession from the hospital saying that the patient is poor. A patient would die of negligence from a doctor, and the court orders compensation calculated on the basis of his age and what he would have earned if he was alive for his expected age of living. Then should the doctor charge the patients depending on their income and future income he is going to earn because his life is saved by the surgery?

There are no straight forward answers to all these questions. Here the dilemma is not like, "Which refrigerator to buy?" It is between right and wrong. Right or wrong are both relative things conceptualized by the human mind, most of the time, to protect the interests of an individual or a group. Both are contextual and perspective based.

Individually when a decision has to be made, one of the ways I suggest is to simply don the role in a particular situation and play it to perfection. A doctor who has admitted his mother to a hospital is in a dilemma whether to give consent for surgery, which is high-risk. He has to simply play the role of a son, not a doctor, for that particular decision.

"When in doubt, identify and play your role in that situation, consequences are immaterial," summarized Resource and packed up his briefcase, bidding me a bye.

Communications

Interaction between two or more people. Communication between body and mind using sensors and intellect. Communication between individuals using sensory and motor organs. I am grasping through sight, sound, touch, taste, and smell, responding through languages of speech, text, body language, and mind—communication between the INERGY and the cosmos through connectivity by meditation.

Time

The most curious and complex dimension of life. "The

topic of Time is too complex and subtle. I will discuss only in relation to health," I insisted. The clock time, The biological time, The mind time. "Your time is as precious as mine. My time is limited. I have to return to the US next week. Go on," he said.

"Time is the dimension in which our lives are etched. Nothing can be erased. It is a one-way lane. It is the only one equal to all. All our activities take place in the realm of time. Date of birth and date of expiry is in time. You wake up at a particular time, work for some time, and go to bed at a particular time. The success of your event depends on the timing, and all the work should be done within a timeline.

'All this TIME,' which is simply rolling ahead in clocks and calendars, relentlessly is just one aspect of time. But there is one more TIME, which is ticking in our brain/ pineal gland, and in all our cells, which determines the lifespan of each cell. There is a concept called 'apoptosis' or 'timed-cell-death.' That means each cell has got its own life span and has to die at a designated time to keep us healthy. If this process goes wrong, and the cells refuse to die and continue to grow, it is called cancer.

Our immune systems will be taking care of these rebellious cells on a day to day basis. If that fails, cancer progresses, is one of the concepts in cancer genesis.

Aging is nothing but the cells and tissues are tuned to our biological clock and progress accordingly. The biological clock is synced to the worldly clock. But it is also maintained by the INERGY, and malfunctioning can cause premature aging.

All our physiological activities are timed. If you sleep late, your digestion gets upset. If your time zone changes suddenly, what is called 'jet lag,' it will take some time to adjust your biological clock to outside time.

There is one more TIME, which is a concept inside our minds. My time, your time, no time to do so many things, time is not passing, time management falls into this category of time, etc. This time is the gap between the thoughts.

If too many thoughts are bombarding you, you have less

time and vice versa. So, if you want to create more time, all you have to do is to reduce the number of thoughts your mind is releasing. This is done by avoiding adding unnecessary thoughts into your data bank from where they are released.

Prioritize your works and execute them slowly and patiently one after the other. Then your thought processes are also well-coordinated with enough time at your disposal. Similarly, when you are locked down at home for many days, create a greater number of useful physical activities. Your mind will be occupied by a number of thoughts released; you will not know when the time has passed.

In the worldly time, which is determined by the rotation of the earth in relation to the sun, we've got only limited time. How well we use it to have a wholesome experience of life with no regrets at the time of the final call is up to us. We have to plan it as a return journey, to face the ultimate reality, happily," I concluded.

I further added, "Worldly time, a rotating wheel: manage well for a wholesome experience of life and death. Biological time is ticking away. Don't meddle with it."

"Mental time: manage your thought process smoothly, to create or kill time," Resource summed up in his usual style.

He looked up his mobile for the message he received some time back.

"Time is up. Thanks for finishing on time. I don't know when I will meet you again," he said and left.

Shirin, who landed here from the US yesterday, was quarantined for some viral infection. Just now, I got a message that she has been shifted to ICU. He left without a word and left me gasping for a word.

Next three weeks, Lockdown was announced. Everyone holed up in their nests. Resource was untraceable.

Has some invisible force added extra free time to most of the people, deducted from a few others' lives? IT employees were the most affected. Their workload from home increased. Freebies like coffee, lunch, etc. disappeared. Weekend shopping and entertainment disappeared. Trees started breathing, and peacocks were dancing inside the city. Police were struggling to impose house arrest for the whole country. It was a painful period for many and revelation for a few.

It was a 'loss-loss' situation for all, but a must-win situation for the human species against an invisible species. It was a lifetime experience for all — when all din was settling, Resource, like God, appeared from nowhere. He was clean-shaven, including his head.

Resource, in his new avatar, declared:

"It was untimely, but as we were discussing in our last meeting, the 'date of expiry' seems to be already printed at the time of 'date of manufacturing.'"

Who was Shirin to me?

Where was she born?

Where was she brought up?

Why is she cremated here?! "It was as per her wishes."

Tears were flowing from my eyes, even though I had not met her, but his expressions were totally blank.

Resource was wondering – "In spite of keeping all healthy habits and being fit, why did she die? What is the meaning of it?"

"Life and death are not two separate entities and not opposite of each other, though they are opposite sides of the same coin. Healthy does not mean that you will live longer." I countered.

Then he nodded, "Die, you must, at least, live healthy and happy" and continued with his story.

"After our divorce a year ago, she had joined a spiritual group in India. She had a longing to settle down in India, but I was not able to help her, as we had divorced. I cremated her according to Hindu rituals as per her last wish. She promised to be with me in her next birth. Hmm...."

I was sobbing, but he was stable. Resource laughed loudly, opened up both his arms, embraced me, and what! He is soft and melting in my arms...

DEATH!!!

Disappeared! Dissolved into me! Did he die? DIE? WHAT IS DEATH?

HOW CAN SEKHAR, THE SOURCE, ANSWER THIS ONE, HE IS YET TO EXPERIENCE? IF HE EXPERIENCES, HE WILL NOT BE THERE TO ANSWER! LET ME GET THE ANSWER FROM 'RESOURCE' WHO HAS DISSOLVED INTO ME.

Hey! Resource! Now it's time for you to explain what is 'DEATH.'

He Started Narrating:

I never died because I was never born. I was your creation, a mental creation, and intellectual interpretation and physical experience.

Don't ask me any questions. I know all your doubts and confusion as I am now inside your mind. I will not explain. I will make you experience death! You are damn scared, aren't you? You will have a pleasant experience.

What Is Happening To Me?

------ My body is changing, my scalp is slowly getting filled up with hair, that too all black!

------ The wrinkles are disappearing; I am celebrating my sixtieth birthday with my family and friends.

135

------ That is Nandu, my second son's, Upanayana.

------ I am sitting in my old clinic.

------ That is Iran, Tehran; Shantaram is explaining how the house we rented in Ilam, that border town, was flattened by Iraqi's bombing just after we vacated it.

------ Oh, nice to see that young couple in their wedding attire with excitement in their eyes. Very, very familiar faces, zoom in. Wow! It's Chandrika and Me!

------ Hostel day at Kurnool, Pradeeps, Bhaskar', Mohans, Ganesh, Ramu, Gopi, Shiv, Mahesh, trying to recognize each. Dr. Haranath, the principal, smiling. ------- That boy in his teens playing with Nagesh, Venu; it's Me? I thought I was more handsome! ------ Rajasree is teaching me, Jamuna is complaining to my mother about our younger brother Ravi. Must be Malathi and Uma! Trying to carry me from the temple back home, too heavy for my age.

------Who is that trying to push me, squeezing me from my warm water world. Somebody's holding me by my feet upside down and beating me on my bums. I was so happy inside, now why are they making me cry, and they are all enjoying it. But I will still smile once this pain subsides. I am feeling something in my stomach, something they are putting in my mouth, the stomach is getting filled, feeling nice, sounds! Light! Warmth! A soothing touch! Taste!

------ I became so tiny, tinier and tinier. I can't feel anything.

I disappeared; where am I? Who am I?

What am I ?...I?... I?

Feeling light, Serene, calm, peace, happiness, blissful

------, boring, no excitement, sweets! Want to taste; no nice smell; no colors, no shapes, no movements; want to see; want that electrifying, exciting experience with the other body!!! Body??? Where is my body??? Resource, why are you torturing me? You are projecting all my memories and feelings, but ... want to eat something delicious, new tastes,

------- want to see, want to really see something new, beautiful, not the same things you are showing.... Music, drums, guitar, veena, flute, so many instruments, orchestra?

Dance rock and roll, Bharatanatyam, Kuchipudi, tribal dance to the drum beats, want to dance! Want my body. What have you done to my body? All these feelings, want to experience one by one, no, all at a time! Ok, one by one. But where is my body? Yes, I want to see it! Sure, I want to see it! ---- Oh! No! Why are people surrounding that body and crying? Why is it not responding? -- What are they doing? Why are they pushing the body into the fire? So merciless! So cruel! No!
Want my body back....

ALL THESE SENSATIONS ARE TORTURING ME TO ENJOY, SO MUCH I HAD MISSED OUT, NOW MY BODY IS BURNT TO ASHES AND THROWN INTO FLOWING WATER!

I want a body. I want to eat; I am so hungry? I want to dance to the music! I had not seen 99.999% of the world!

And the body is destroyed. Want to meet, mate! No! I can't control it! Can't tolerate this torture! These desires, these cravings are haunting me. Without a body, how can I douse these fires of desires?

They are burning me. I can't enjoy it, I can't suppress, I can't sleep to forget, and I can't even die! Already dead! This is HELL!

Yes, this is hell! HELL!!! HELL!!! HELL .to hell with you. What? Have I created this HELL? But HOW? Oh, with my own desires (unfulfilled) at the time of death? But I didn't know that I would die, no, I knew but not so soon it will come! But please, please, I want my body. I can't tolerate this HELL anymore!

What! You want to take me back further, to show me what all things I did for others? You want to show me all my thoughts without the intellect supporting me, my nasty thoughts? My selfish thoughts? My cunning thoughts?

You mean to say I will start all these again, once I get back one more body? No, no, no...enough is enough. Don't show me further. I am already in the torture chamber of my unending desires... I don't want anything more. Please, Raja, Resource, I helped you so much. Stop this nonsense. You can't? Because I have created it!

Then get me a body. What? I have to wait in this hell for more time. My God! Where is God? I want to pray to him. He won't see me!

OK, I want a body, please search for one. Do I have to choose? I have a choice? You will guide me. OK. If I want to fulfill all my existing desires, I have to choose a womb from a family where all these are possible but not guaranteed.

And once you get that, you will not have control over your desires. They will become unending passions and haunt you in hell. If you choose differently, you will get a body and environment to help you in controlling and slowly dissolving the desires...the choice is yours.

Tell me I will start searching for a future body for you. But once you take your body, you will forget about hell, death. And all your memories will only become your nature and just roll you down that path of bodily pleasures, and you will forget about yourself and get identified with the body. Decide now.'

Ok! I can't wait long in this hell, where I can't even meet the god of death. Nobody except you is haunting me with my own thoughts and threatening me with exposing my whole past! A reasonably decent body will do. Go! Don't waste time! I can't even count time here!

Ok, thanks, bye. I am entering into that future body.

OH! They are naming my cute body. Rajasekhar! What? There is no other name in this world! Ok, what is the name? I will manage it. Make me grow fast. Fast forward. Again, you are with me. Again, that monkey! Principal! Srinivasarao, Sesha. Same old story. University first in my class, same old competition, Entrance test, Complications of surgeries, Iran, Snowfall delaying flight to India with wife and two small kids, struggling to get a foothold in Bangalore. I know all these at least from now onwards.

Why have you brought me back to the same old story?

"Hey! Resource, were you sleeping?"

You didn't die. I only took into a flashback as far as I could. What you experienced was between your last death and this birth, the hell as you felt.

Now I began understanding about death and after death. Death is the remnants of our memories of unfulfilled desires after the body perishes. As we try to fulfill all our desires before death, we end up with more and more. They become our tormentors and force us to beg for a body, again to follow the unending cycles of birth and death.

So, if we want to enjoy the bliss and peace after the body dissipates, we must not have memories of desires. To achieve that, we must start detachment from the fruits of our actions, which are nothing but our desires.

The path looks simple. But hardly anybody is able to achieve it. Why???

I was jolted by Satya, "Sekhar! Rajasekhar! Everybody has left. Hurry!"

I just opened my eyes from probably my longest meditation of my life, with Majestic, mystical Mount Kailash in front and divine Lake Manasarovar behind in the mighty Himalayan range of mountains.

Was this whole story a culmination to my wandering mind about health and disease and struggling intellect to find answers?

Does Shirin represent the uncertainties of life? RESOURCE (mind) dissolving in SOURCE (Intellect) to create "Happiness energy." Health?

Raja dissolved into Sekhar!

"Rajasekhar started moving!

Still, it is the beginning of our Parikrama (circumambulation). "Long way to go!" Satya Prakash started almost pulling me behind him.

Started moving chanting, "Om Namah Shivaya."

Became breathless on the way, stopped a while, and leaned onto my walking stick for rest, as advised by my guide on tour, Mr. Srinivas Reddy, a veteran of Himalayan adventures. Some of them moving ahead, some retiring, I was just looking at the mountain far away, smiling at my fate.

Somebody tapped on my back. A long-bearded man of almost my age, with a turban around his head, with an infectious smile on his face, with some followers behind him, whispered into my ears; "book on Health or hell" is ok. Foundation is done; the building of careers outlined. But who is guiding you? Whom are you teaching?

By the time I could come to my senses, he had already gone far off. And we should not hurry or run during high altitude trekking, Murali, the leader, had advised me at the beginning of our journey.

So, I just started wondering. "WHO?"

Not an END

Congrats on going through this book. Now you have got the information about health. Convert into knowledge pearls by repeating the 'Ten Commandments' at least thrice a day and get wisdom out of it by critically analyzing it and implementing it.

"You have paid for it, now encash it as Health."

PART B

THE MANTRA

This mantra is for people who have read this book and want to practice and Identify with the INERGY, by reciting and repeating the following verse:

"I am INERGY, which is intelligence driven energy. I am made of happiness, made of peace, I am eternal. I am not this body. This body is mine. It is only a gadget for my usage. I am INERGY, intelligence guided cosmic energy. I am eternal. I have no birth or death. I am permanent. I have taken this body to experience life. I have to maintain the body, but I am not this body."
All the pleasures and sufferings are only for the body. I, being INERGY, is only a witness. I am made of happiness and peace and so I am always happy.
I am happiness. I am peace. I am bliss."

Those who have 'no time' to go through the whole book, can at least get some benefit from this mantra.

Scan this QR code and listen to this mantra, earphones recommended to get the feel of yourself as peace and happiness.

PART C

NECTAR
1
WHAT IS HEALTH?

- Health is an expression of life. Synchrony of physical process, chemical process, energy, and intelligence.
- Health is not a destination but a part of the journey of life.
- The physical process of life can be understood as the hardware part of a computer.
- The chemical process is like the source and distribution of power for the functioning of the system.
- The energy process of life is the software part of the system.
- The intelligence process is the operating system downloaded from the Web of Cosmic Intelligence.
- 'Inergy,' is the intelligence guided energy that drives the Physico-chemical processes of life.
- The brain is like the Central Processing Unit.

BEACON (1)

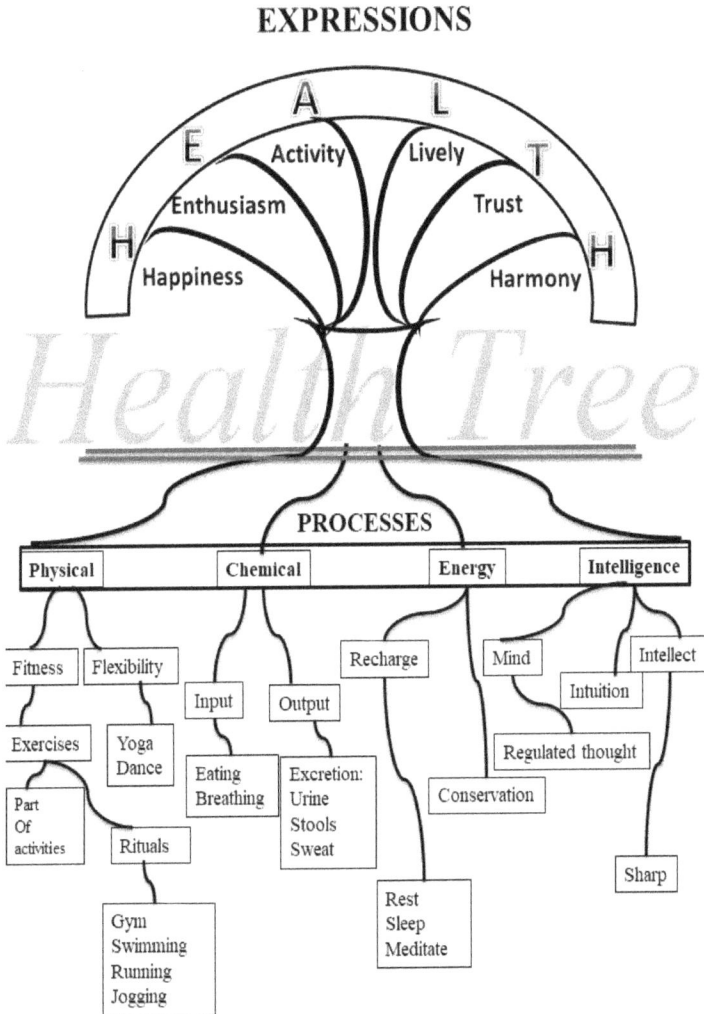

NECTAR
2
WHY HEALTH?

Health is the unseen foundation for building any career in life.

- All the dreams of future collapse if there is a major health issue.
- The economic status of individuals, families, and societies are adversely affected by problems of health.
- Health is the only issue where all the nations are on one platform, irrespective of their different ideologies.
- We always take health for granted until it is affected.
- Health is more than wealth and is the essential ingredient to experience wholesome life.

BEACON (2)

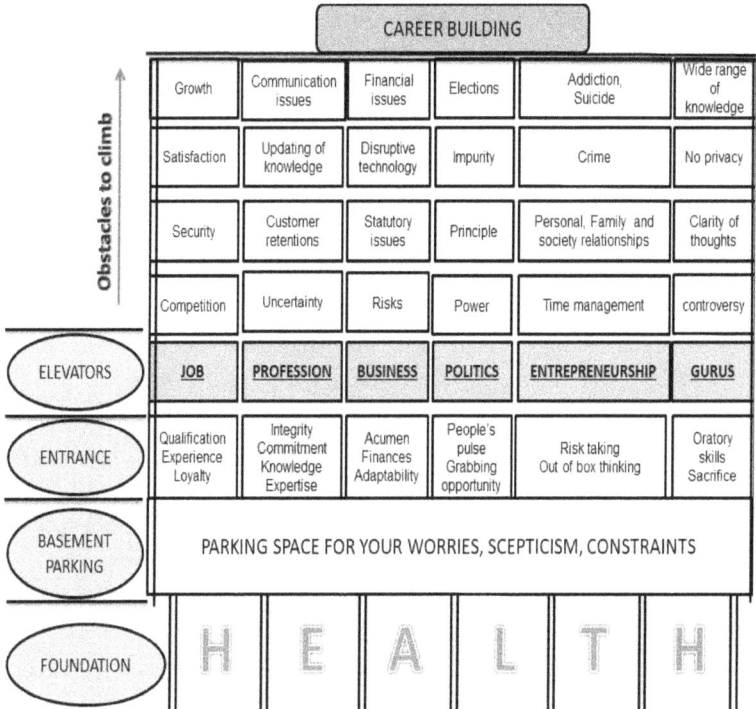

CAREER BUILDING					
Growth	Communication issues	Financial issues	Elections	Addiction, Suicide	Wide range of knowledge
Satisfaction	Updating of knowledge	Disruptive technology	Impurity	Crime	No privacy
Security	Customer retentions	Statutory issues	Principle	Personal, Family and society relationships	Clarity of thoughts
Competition	Uncertainty	Risks	Power	Time management	controversy
JOB	**PROFESSION**	**BUSINESS**	**POLITICS**	**ENTREPRENEURSHIP**	**GURUS**
Qualification Experience Loyalty	Integrity Commitment Knowledge Expertise	Acumen Finances Adaptability	People's pulse Grabbing opportunity	Risk taking Out of box thinking	Oratory skills Sacrifice

Obstacles to climb (left axis, arrow up)

ELEVATORS · ENTRANCE · BASEMENT PARKING · FOUNDATION

PARKING SPACE FOR YOUR WORRIES, SCEPTICISM, CONSTRAINTS

HEALTH

NECTAR
3
HOW TO BE HEALTHY?

Disturbances in the life processes by external or internal forces lead to deterioration in health.

- External factors like accidents, wars, natural disasters, and epidemics may not be under our control. But even there, the fittest and the healthiest survive.
- Most of the chronic diseases are caused by negligence in the maintenance of health by inappropriate lifestyles and ignorance.
- Myths and misplaced priorities in the maintenance of health are the leading cause of all the diseases.
- The seed of disease is sown in mind through the disturbed and disorganized thought processes.
- The explosion of unwanted thoughts result in disturbances in Physico-chemical processes of life and are diagnosed as diseases.
- Physical and chemical processes can treat diseases. But they can be cured, prevented, or reversed only through the management of the Inergy.

BEACON (3)

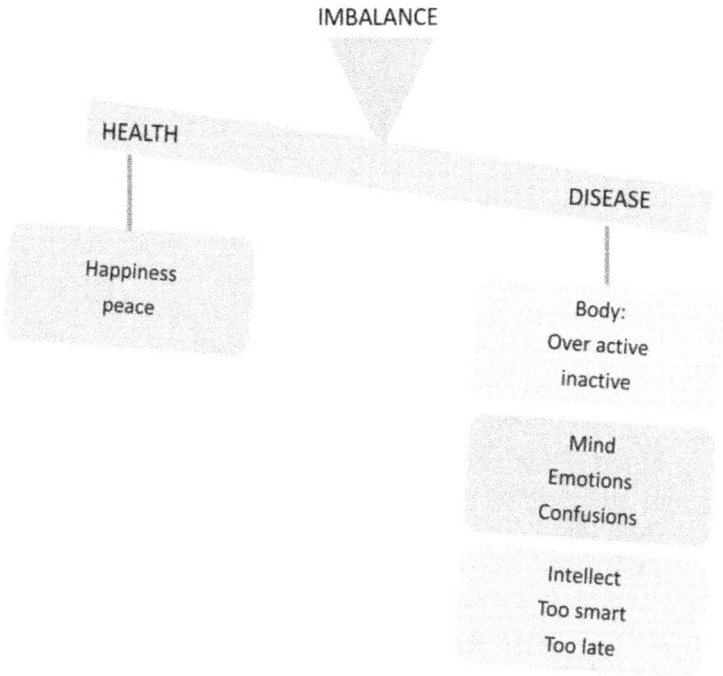

NECTAR
4
WHEN TO INTERFERE?

- Any intervention in treatment is to be decided by the patient. If the patient can't decide, then the attendant's main goal is to ease the suffering of the patient and ensure longevity.
- Minor issues can be diagnosed by consciously observing the signals from the sensors in the body. They can be managed by individuals by home remedies and simple measures.
- Persistent minor issues can be tackled by a family physician or a general practitioner at leisure.
- Significant issues like bleeding, unexplained loss of body weight, weakness, and mental disturbances are to be addressed as a priority.
- Emergencies like change in consciousness, accidents, severe pain, imbalance in posture or speech, etc. are to be attended immediately at the nearest big hospital.
- To stop treatment for any patient, the individual must take the call after discussing it with his doctor and his close people as it may have repercussions.

BEACON (4)

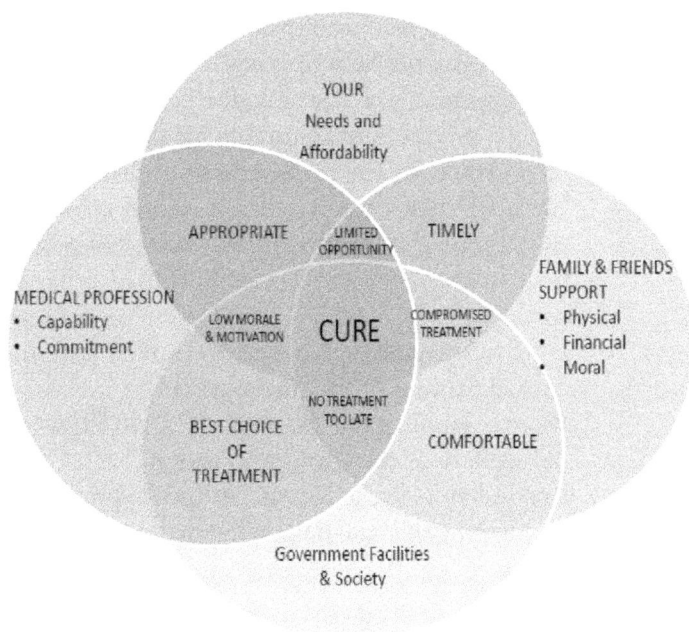

YOUR
Needs and
Affordability

APPROPRIATE   LIMITED OPPORTUNITY   TIMELY

MEDICAL PROFESSION
- Capability
- Commitment

LOW MORALE & MOTIVATION   CURE   COMPROMISED TREATMENT

FAMILY & FRIENDS SUPPORT
- Physical
- Financial
- Moral

BEST CHOICE OF TREATMENT   NO TREATMENT TOO LATE   COMFORTABLE

Government Facilities & Society

NECTAR
5
WHO AM I?

- You have to take responsibility for your health, and others can only help or guide.
- Government is responsible for health care policies.
- Public, private, and charitable medical institutes are responsible for the management of diseases.
- NGOs, Yoga centers, fitness centers, meditation centers, religious and spiritual gurus can guide and help in the management of health in a particular society.
- Environmentalists, nature lovers take part in the overall process of life management.
- World organizations like WHO, UNICEF work for the welfare of the world population.
- But individually, it is your attitude, approach, and philosophy that will help in the maintenance of your health.

BEACON (5)

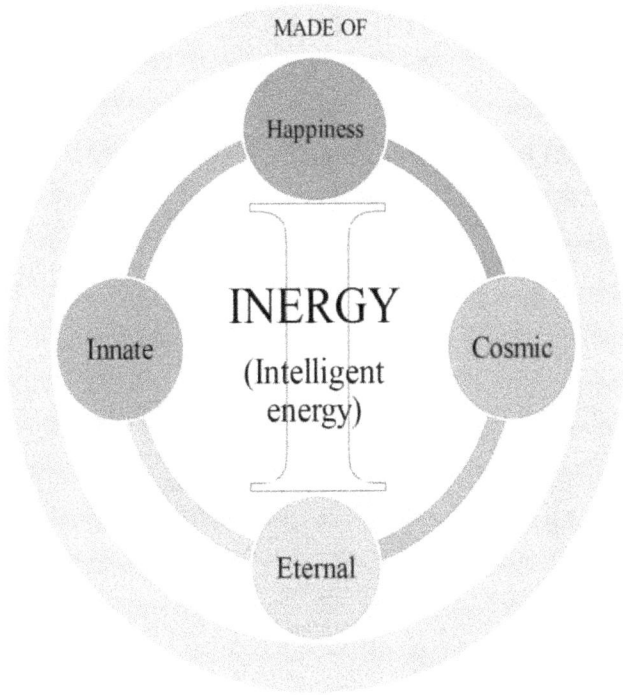

NECTAR
6
WHERE TO GO WHEN DISEASED?

- Diagnosis or knowing which part of the system is affected, and what has affected it is the initial step. A qualified doctor is required for this.
- A minor ailment of short duration is to be first attended by a qualified family physician or general practitioner from any system of medicine, in which you have faith.
- The attending doctor has to attempt to confirm the cause of the disease and treat it, along with treatment of the symptoms, if any.
- For a complete diagnosis, a process of history taking, clinical examination, investigations through laboratory or imaging (radiology), and plan the treatment. A specialist may be involved during this if needed.
- Any long-term disease is better treated at a stand-alone specialty center, like an eye hospital, orthopedic hospital, etc.
- Emergencies and major life-threatening illnesses and multi-system diseases are to be treated at the nearby bigger hospitals like teaching hospitals, multi-specialty hospitals.
- The choice of the treating doctor depends on expertise, experience, and humanity. You should feel comfortable with the doctor.
- Your trust in the doctor and the doctor's commitment to your well-being are very crucial in the treatment. The doctor-patient relationship should be more than a service provider-consumer relationship.

- You can opt for the second opinion only if there is no clarity or deficit of trust. Multiple opinions will cause more confusion and delay in treatment.

BEACON (6)

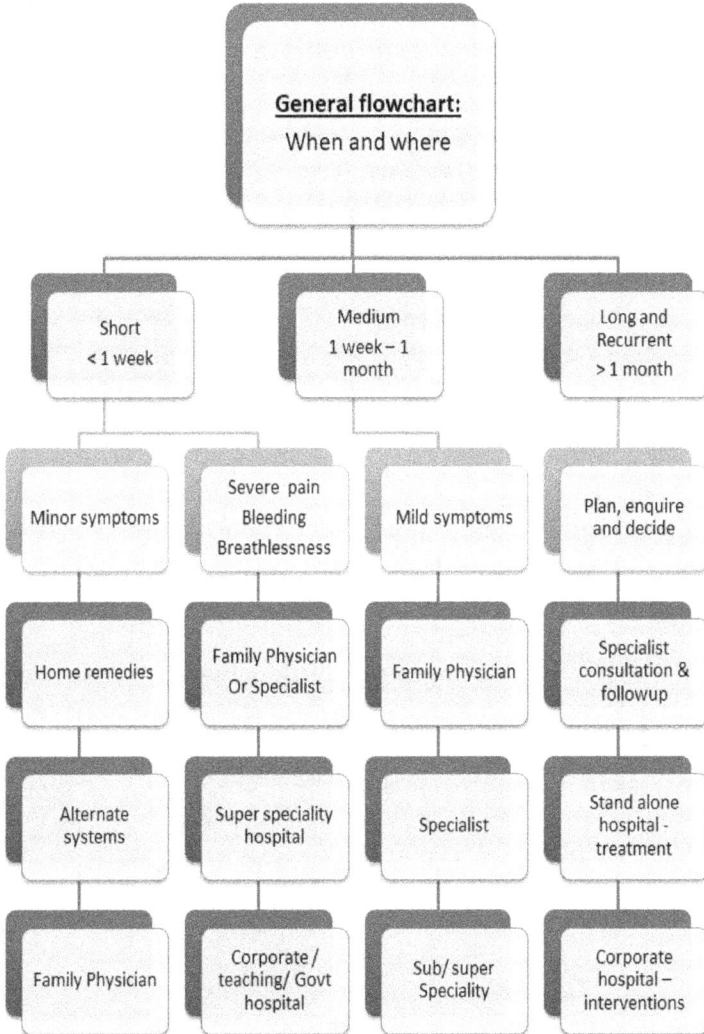

NECTAR
7
WHICH WAY FORWARD?

- You are the 'Inergy,' and the intelligence guided energy that drives your body.
- Your body is the physical part, and the actions of it are through chemical processes.
- Your body is only a sophisticated machine and requires proper maintenance. It has a shelf life, date of manufacturer, and date of expiry.
- You are made of happiness and peace and are eternal.
- You experience your life using your body, through the thoughts generated by your mind and intellect.
- Every individual life is nothing but their thoughts(data), released from the mind (databank), created from repeated actions coupled with emotions.
- The limited identity creates emotions with the body and its extensions like name, fame, position, relationships, etc.
- If your life is to be happy, peaceful, useful, and purposeful, then you have to get happy, peaceful, useful, and purposeful thoughts stored in your mind.
- To create a thought bank consisting of these types of thoughts, your actions should be such. Do every work happily, peacefully, usefully, and with a purpose.
- A happy, peaceful, useful, and purposeful life manifests health.

BEACON (7)

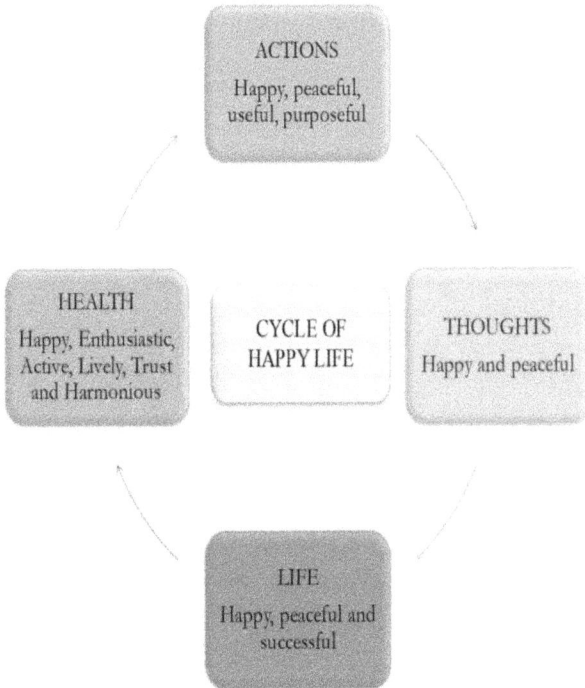

ACTIONS
Happy, peaceful, useful, purposeful

HEALTH
Happy, Enthusiastic, Active, Lively, Trust and Harmonious

CYCLE OF HAPPY LIFE

THOUGHTS
Happy and peaceful

LIFE
Happy, peaceful and successful

SELF ASSESSMENT OF YOUR KNOWLEDGE

1. If you feel you are perfectly healthy, what will be your priority in life?

Feeling healthy, it's a very subjective matter, and most of us believe that if specific known parameters like BP, sugar, and body weight are normal, then we are healthy. But that is only partly true. Physical or chemical parameters do not merely measure health. There are different indicators of health. There is also mental health that needs to be taken care of. My first and foremost priority will always be health. Taking care of it is a routine and continuous process. Once I feel I am in top form, I will work on a hobby or a passion project to keep myself happy. This, of course, is beside my day-job.

2. If you are diagnosed with a 'lifetime disease (e.g., Diabetes, Hypertension, increased cholesterol), what changes would you like to make in your career?

Almost all lifestyle diseases are reversible in their early stages. So instead of making changes in our careers, we must change our mindset. Collect all the information about the condition from a reliable source like your family physician, discuss it with your family/well-wishers. Introspect and analyze the source and take corrective measures. Your aim is not to manage or treat the disease, but to get rid of it permanently. But don't postpone starting a treatment or doing required investigations, thinking that if you start treatment, it will be permanent. You can't wish away your disease or cure it by will power. The process of reversing the disease takes perseverance, patience, and faith. It is not magical. It's by practicing a higher level of living, which yields many benefits, including the reversal of diseases. This process, once developed, happiness and peace are guaranteed. (would help to give one or two tips)

3. If you are a smoker/drinker, and your father and uncle have lived for more than 90 years, despite those habits, what is your take on that?

Quitting smoking or alcohol is not merely preventing or treating a disease. You may want to do it for better health, yes. The real reason you should quit is that: you don't want to be dependent on it. You can proudly say that I have quit because I didn't want to be a slave.

4. Is being healthy the only purpose of our life?

Being healthy is not a purpose or destination. It is your journey. It's part of you. It is the basis of your life on which you can build your dreams and enjoy the fruits of your actions. Health is your right and responsibility.

5. Your parents have diabetes, and so how do you think you can prevent it?

If both your parents have diabetes, there is a higher chance of you getting diabetes. Statistically, many people who are in that category are obese with a careless lifestyle.

When I ask them, their standard reply is, anyway I am going to get diabetes as it is in my genes. So, I want to enjoy life, eat all varieties of sweets before it catches up with me.

This is a defeatist attitude. Though their chances are high, they are more likely to be from similar attitudes and lifestyles than genes. If it was purely genetic, your parents should have got it from their birth or childhood.

You have an opportunity to prevent it or at least postpone it by following certain principles in life. The most important thing is to remove the concept that eating is the most essential part of enjoying life.

6. What are all the gadgets (Example: step counter, calorie calculator, and body fat measurement equipment) you want to get to get rid of your obesity?

The single most important gadget is your mindset. If you have a proper understanding of obesity, the role of diet, exercises, planning, and execution, you don't need any other gadget. A simple weighing machine will do. All you need to do is follow these four rules.

1. Identify and accept obesity as a disease.
2. Decide to get rid of it.
3. Plan it like it's the most important project of your life.
4. Start implementing the project NOW.

7. Which system of treatment (Example: Ayurveda, allopathy, naturopathy, homeopathy) you follow, and why?

There are many misconceptions like modern medicine have side effects, and alternate systems do not, which is false. Modern medicine investigates and notes down all the side effects, and the other networks will try to gloss over them. Every system has its advantages and disadvantages. Choose them properly. Read about the methods from credible sources and talk to experts before you make a choice.

*ANY SYSTEM YOU FOLLOW SHOULD NOT BE DEPENDENT ON YOUR BIASED OR HALF-BAKED KNOWLEDGE OR EMOTIONAL OR RELIGIOUS BELIEFS.

8. Your wife noticed a painless swelling in her left breast for the past two months. Your son appears for final year exams in 1 month. When do you want her to go to a doctor for a consultation?

Any abnormal swellings, mostly if painless, consult your

family physician at the earliest. Get it thoroughly diagnosed, and treatment options can be decided depending on the seriousness of the disease. If the doctor says it needs further investigations like mammography or biopsy, then don't delay it because it will be excluded. Any cancer, the earlier it is diagnosed and treated, the better are the results. Early intervention is the most critical factor in the cure of any disease. Her sisters or siblings may also have to be examined. Insist on that. Learn to prioritize things.

9. Your 15-year-old daughter has got a mole on her face for ten years now, and she thinks she's ugly. How soon will you get the surgery done?

A mole on the face of a young girl for more than a decade excludes an acute disease from a medical point of view. However, talk to your daughter about body-image issues and preferably get her to see a counselor.

10. You have been bleeding during passing stools for two months. The doctor has advised a procedure to cure it. You want to get it done after you return from your assignment in the US for one year. What factors do you consider?

Some age-old notions like bleeding with stools are from 'body heat,' or because of eating a particular food or drinking coffee, etc. Even though they may be partly true, there is no way one can exclude disease as a cause of bleeding, especially cancer of the anal canal or rectum. If a diagnosis of 'piles' as the cause of bleeding is made, it's better to get it cured and go abroad than waiting for one year, by which time it might progress.

11. In your village, you want to start a charity neuro hospital for the local people, and you want to give them all the imported medical equipment you had to improve their health. But they are skeptical. What will you do?

Most of the time, we decide what the people want, instead

of letting them decide what they need. We try to donate what we have rather than what they seek. If your people need good hygienic food, then give them that food and also teach them. Provide them with a water filtration plant rather than a neuro hospital. Also, education so they can gain employment and skills.

12. Your brother is a world-renowned microbiologist settled in Geneva. You want him to produce vaccines against all possible diseases. He says it's not impossible but simply laughs at your idea. Why?

Diseases caused by microbes are only a small part of the health issue. A human being is capable of harming himself by simply overeating, taking drugs, violence in the name of religion. If there is a vaccine to give us sanity, it is most welcome.

13. There is an outbreak of Typhoid every summer in your neighborhood slum. Doctors and pharmaceutical companies conduct free health camps and distribute free medicines, along with some clubs. What is your suggestion?

Typhoid is a transmissible disease caused by a particular bacterium. It spreads by contaminated water or food. Get to the source of the illness by investigating or checking water supplied or food sourced. It can be permanently prevented.

14. My ex- patient's father in law has a lot of bleeding after passing stools. He is in a city 600 kilometers away. She wants to shift him to my new hospital. What was my advice?

If the patient is suffering from excessive bleeding anywhere in the body or for any reason, he/she should be taken to the nearest hospital to assess the nature and severity of bleeding, before taking any further decision.

15. My neighbour brings her husband to me with

severe chest pain and says, you have cured my father with a similar complaint. Though you are a 'proctologist', I want you to treat my husband. I don't trust anybody. What should I do?

Any chest pain, we divide it into cardiac or noncardiac origin first. It shows the importance of not missing any heart attack as a cause of chest pain as it can be fatal if not treated immediately. So an ECG to exclude a heart attack is a must before deciding on who and where to treat. Patients' faith in us should not make us overconfident and harm them.

16. You were trekking and had an injury with bleeding, taken to a clinic nearby. He suggests wound suturing to stop bleeding. But you want a plastic surgeon to do the job.

If suturing has to be done to control bleeding from a wound, it should be done at the nearest place. Plastic surgical corrections can be done later if required.

ABOUT THE AUTHOR

As I started pondering over the authorship, I realized that I am only the writer, and at best, a compiler, but the authority to write is not mine alone. It has arisen from the anxiety, ignorance, doubts, dilemmas, leading to questions put forward by you, a collective representative of thousands of my patients. The extract of my answers is from some of my patients/relatives and my colleagues' behavior. The churning process of the emotions and intellect was done by the diseases on one side and the health on the other side. The resultant cream is this book. So, I consider you the author.

For further clarifications, practicing methods, online interactions with Dr. Rajasekhar you can visit our website below or even find us on other social media platforms.

🌐 www.ChiragHospital.in

f @chiraghospitals 📷 dr.rajasekhar.mysore

✉ doctorrajasekharmysore@gmail.com

☎ +919353780276

▶ https://www.youtube.com/channel/UCGA6onwllA dBy6_hA4nanNw

www.ingramcontent.com/pod-product-compliance
Lightning Source LLC
Chambersburg PA
CBHW022107280326
41933CB00007B/296